Population Health

Editors

DEVDUTTA G. SANGVAI
ANTHONY J. VIERA

PRIMARY CARE:
CLINICS IN OFFICE PRACTICE

www.primarycare.theclinics.com

Consulting Editor
JOEL J. HEIDELBAUGH

December 2019 • Volume 46 • Number 4

ELSEVIER

1600 John F. Kennedy Boulevard • Suite 1800 • Philadelphia, Pennsylvania, 19103-2899

http://www.theclinics.com

PRIMARY CARE: CLINICS IN OFFICE PRACTICE Volume 46, Number 4
December 2019 ISSN 0095-4543, ISBN-13: 978-0-323-67890-2

Editor: Jessica McCool
Developmental Editor: Laura Fisher

Primary Care: Clinics in Office Practice (ISSN: 0095-4543) is published quarterly by Elsevier Inc., 360 Park Avenue South, New York, NY 10010-1710. Months of issue are March, June, September, and December. Periodicals postage paid at New York, NY and additional mailing offices. Subscription prices are $246.00 per year (US individuals), $505.00 (US institutions), $100.00 (US students), $303.00 (Canadian individuals), $572.00 (Canadian institutions), $175.00 (Canadian students), $357.00 (international individuals), $572.00 (international institutions), and $175.00 (international students). Foreign air speed delivery is included in all *Clinics* subscription prices. All prices are subject to change without notice. POSTMASTER: Send address changes to *Primary Care: Clinics in Office Practice*, Elsevier Periodicals Customer Service, 11830 Westline Industrial Drive, St. Louis, MO 63146. Customer Service Health Sciences Division, Subscription Customer Service, 3251 Riverport Lane, Maryland Heights, MO 63043. **Customer Service: 1-800-654-2452 (U.S. and Canada); 314-447-8871 (outside U.S. and Canada). Fax: 314-447-8029. E-mail: journalscustomerservice-usa@elsevier.com (for print support); journalsonlinesupport-usa@elsevier.com (for online support).**

Reprints. For copies of 100 or more, of articles in this publication, please contact the Commercial Reprints Department, Elsevier Inc., 360 Park Avenue South, New York, NY 10010-1710. Tel. 212-633-3874; Fax: 212-633-3820; E-mail: reprints@elsevier.com.

Primary Care: Clinics in Office Practice is covered in *MEDLINE/PubMed (Index Medicus)* and *EMBASE/Excerpta Medica, Current Contents/Clinical Medicine, and ISI/BIOMED.*

Contributors

CONSULTING EDITOR

JOEL J. HEIDELBAUGH, MD, FAAFP, FACG
Clinical Professor, Departments of Family Medicine and Urology, University of Michigan Medical School, Ann Arbor, Michigan

EDITORS

DEVDUTTA G. SANGVAI, MD, MBA
Assistant Professor, Department of Family Medicine and Community Health, Pediatrics and Psychiatry, Duke University Medical Center, Associate Chief Medical Officer, Duke University Health System, Medical Director of DukeWELL, Durham, North Carolina

ANTHONY J. VIERA, MD, MPH
Professor and Chair, Department of Family Medicine and Community Health, Duke University, Durham, North Carolina

AUTHORS

JOHN B. ANDERSON, MD, MPH
Chief Medical Officer, Duke Primary Care; Assistant Professor, Department of Family and Community Medicine, Duke University Health System, Durham, North Carolina

SCOTT A. BERKOWITZ, MD, MBA
Associate Professor of Medicine, Division of Cardiology, Senior Medical Director, Accountable Care, Executive Director, Johns Hopkins Medicine Alliance for Patients, Baltimore, Maryland

L. EBONY BOULWARE, MD
Professor, Departments of Medicine, Community and Family Medicine, and Population Health Sciences, Duke University, Durham, North Carolina

THERESA M. COLES, PhD
Assistant Professor, Department of Population Health Sciences, Duke University, Durham, North Carolina

SARAH J. CONWAY, MD
Assistant Professor of Medicine, Department of Medicine, Medical Director, Accountable Care, Baltimore, Maryland

LESLEY H. CURTIS, PhD
Professor, Departments of Population Health Sciences and Medicine, Duke Clinical Research Institute, Duke University, Durham, North Carolina

CRAIG E. DEAO, MHA
Managing Director, Studer Group, Pensacola, Florida

DAVID C. DUGDALE, MD
Professor, Division of General Internal Medicine, Department of Medicine, University of Washington School of Medicine, Seattle, Washington

TIMOTHY G. FERRIS, MD, MPH
Massachusetts General Physicians Organization, Department of Medicine, Massachusetts General Hospital, Harvard Medical School, Boston, Massachusetts

ROBERT W. FIELDS, MD, MHA
SVP and CMO Population Health, Mount Sinai Health System, New York, New York; Assistant Professor, The Institute for Family Health

NIYUM GANDHI, BA
Assistant Professor, Health System Design and Global Health, EVP and Chief Population Health Officer, Mount Sinai Health System, New York, New York

RESHMA GUPTA, MD, MSHPM
Medical Director of Quality and Value, UCLA Health, Assistant Professor, Division of General Internal Medicine and Health Services Research, David Geffen School of Medicine, University of California Los Angeles, Los Angeles, California; Co-director of Costs of Care, Inc

JENNIFER HOULIHAN, MSP
Vice President of Value-Based Care & Population Health, Wake Forest Baptist Medical Center, CIN-Population Health, Winston-Salem, North Carolina

STEVE LEFFLER, MD, FACEP
Interim President, Chief Quality and Population Health Officer, University of Vermont Health Network, The University of Vermont Medical Center, Burlington, Vermont

MICHELLE J. LYN, MBA, MHA
Assistant Professor and Chief, Division of Community Health, Duke Department of Family Medicine and Community Health, Duke University, Durham, North Carolina

LEAH M. MARCOTTE, MD
Clinical Assistant Professor, Division of General Internal Medicine, Department of Medicine, University of Washington School of Medicine, Associate Medical Director for Population Health, Seattle, Washington

HEATHER MARSTILLER, MBOE
Associate Vice President of Operations and Performance Excellence, Duke Primary Care, Duke University Health System, Durham, North Carolina

VIVIANA MARTINEZ-BIANCHI, MD, FAAFP
Associate Professor and Family Medicine Residency Program Director, Duke Department of Family Medicine and Community Health, Duke University, Durham, North Carolina

NARAYANA S. MURALI, MD, Dip. NB, CPE, FACP
EVP Care Delivery & Chief Strategy Officer, Marshfield Clinic Health System, Marshfield Clinic, Marshfield, Wisconsin

NICOLE O'CONNOR, MD
Chair, Practice Improvement Team, Lead, Patient Advisory Council, Tufts University Family Medicine Residency, Malden Family Medicine Center, Cambridge Health Alliance, Assistant Professor of Family Medicine, Tufts University School of Medicine, Malden, Massachusetts

MICHAEL PIGNONE, MD, MPH, MACP
Department of Internal Medicine, Dell Medical School, University of Texas, Austin, Texas

SHANA RATNER, MD, FACP
Department of Medicine, Division of General Internal Medicine and Clinical Epidemiology, University of North Carolina Chapel Hill, Chapel Hill, North Carolina

GREGORY SAWIN, MD, MPH
Program Director, Tufts University Family Medicine Residency, Malden Family Medicine Center, Cambridge Health Alliance, Associate Professor of Family Medicine, Tufts University School of Medicine, Instructor Part-Time, Harvard University Faculty of Medicine, Malden, Massachusetts

KEVIN SHAH, MD, MBA
Associate Chief Medical Officer for Innovation and Improvement, Duke Primary Care; Assistant Professor, Department of Medicine, Duke University Health System, Durham, North Carolina

LISA P. SHOCK, DrPH(c), MHS, PA-C
Evolent Health, Vice President, Clinical Strategy & Operations, Value Based Care, Raleigh, North Carolina; Duke University Medical Center, Consulting Faculty, Geriatrics Education Center, Durham, North Carolina; Department of Health Policy & Management, Executive Doctoral Student (DrPH), University of North Carolina, Gillings School of Global Public Health, Chapel Hill, North Carolina

MINA SILBERBERG, PhD
Associate Professor and Vice-Chief for Research and Evaluation, Duke Division of Community Health, Department of Family Medicine and Community Health, Faculty Affiliate, Duke Council on Race and Ethnicity, Duke University, Durham, North Carolina

JASON H. WASFY, MD, MPhil
Cardiology Division, Department of Medicine, Massachusetts General Hospital, Massachusetts General Physicians Organization, Harvard Medical School, Boston, Massachusetts

BERKELEY YORKERY, MPP
Associate Director, North Carolina Institute of Medicine, Morrisville, North Carolina

ADAM J. ZOLOTOR, MD, DrPH
President and CEO, North Carolina Institute of Medicine, Morrisville, North Carolina; Professor of Family Medicine, University of North Carolina Chapel Hill, Chapel Hill, North Carolina

Contents

This article defines population health as the health outcomes of a group of individuals, including the distribution of such outcomes within the group. Population health includes health outcomes, patterns of health determinants, and policies and interventions that link these two. Attention to social and environmental, as well as medical, determinants of health is essential. The population health lens can be used at the individual, practice, institutional, and community levels. The need for primary care to engage in population health stems from the importance of social and environmental factors, the nature of primary care, and contextual changes.

Primary care clinicians care for an extremely diverse range of patients, and they therefore have numerous opportunities to measure and act to improve the health of various populations. In order to take effective actions to improve the health of their patient populations, primary care clinicians must measure health. Strong population health metrics are characterized by their high validity, consistency, feasibility, and interpretability. Population health metrics should be applied longitudinally to obtain the most information from available data. Optimal population health metrics are actionable and facilitate the implementation of effective strategies to improve population health through administrative or clinical programs.

Many health care systems are shifting to value-based care and beginning to integrate population-based strategies into care delivery. Preventive care is an important domain of this work. Properly applied, these services improve population health and reduce health care costs. Preventive care comprises a substantial proportion of quality metrics for which providers are held accountable. This article discusses prevention through a public health lens, highlighting opportunities in ambulatory care settings to collaborate with community-based organizations and community health workers, redefine primary care teams, and design population-based approaches to improve health.

relationships with patients. Smart technology will support these relationships, empower and engage patients, and build confidence that their health care team will take excellent care of them. Investments need to shift from catastrophic hospital-based care to proactive prevention and wellness, pushing us to think of health beyond health care. Systems need to build a culture of continuous improvement, supported by data-driven improvement science, and keep a sharp focus on the patient experience of care.

There is growing recognition that social determinants of health influence individual and population health. A well-designed population health management strategy can yield improved outcomes for a given community, while improving the financial health of health care systems and providers. This article provides an overview of aligned care delivery, community engagement, education, technology, and other key strategies required to address the needs of patients and communities. A holistic vision incorporating social factors can lead to a return on investment and improvement in the health of a community, at the same time decreasing health care costs for the population managed.

The United States spends more per capita on health care than any other country and has worse health outcomes. Public policy can influence almost all aspects of health. Publicly funded insurance pays for health care for more than half of Americans. For individuals and employers that purchase insurance, the regulatory environment influences which insurance products can be purchased as well as by whom and for how much. Health policy levers at federal, state, and local levels can exert financial and regulatory influence over care. This influence determines what is health care, with increasing federal and state efforts to encourage nontraditional services.

Improving population health in a sustainable way requires collaboration within the medical community and also working through partnerships among multiple community and societal stakeholders. One example of stakeholder engagement is engagement of the community whose health will be affected. Stakeholder engagement has benefits for the quality, sustainability, and impact of population health research and interventions. Several principles of engagement have been developed; common elements across these principles are power sharing, respect, humility, colearning, commitment, and a goal of making change. There is a growing pool of resources available to help clinicians enhance their skills in stakeholder engagement.

True population health management cannot be realized by health care systems acting alone, nor by solely delivering high-quality care at lower costs.

Successful models of population health must not myopically focus on care delivery but must also engage partners across their communities to address community culture as well as the broader social determinants of health. Modern models of population health must incorporate both innovation as well as reform in the clinical delivery process. Use of team-based care, targeted population interventions, and creativity in redesigned incentives are core competencies necessary to effectively change the way health care is delivered across populations.

Health care delivery in the United States has become complex and inefficient. With national health care gross domestic product and out-of-pocket expenses increasing, the nation has not yet improved the quality of health care compared with similar nations. As a result, the public asks for greater population health, improved patient experience, and reduced expenses. In this article, the author discuss how key stakeholders, including policy makers, health systems, patients, and employers, understand how these components of health care value are defined, interlink, and provide opportunities for improvement. The author also outlines concrete improvement opportunities from across the country.

American health care is shifting from a fixed-cost, fee-for-service payment model to value-based payment, in which providers including physicians and hospitals increasingly face incentives to reduce the total cost of care and meet specific quality benchmarks. Leaders of organizations that pay for health care and employers have encouraged this shift in response to substantial increases in health care costs and generally mediocre health outcomes compared with other countries. Here, we make the case that although the pace and details of such payment reforms are uncertain, these underlying structural economic challenges make a transition to some sort of value-based care inevitable.

Academic medicine is at an inflection point with the changing priorities of health care to focus more on population health. In this new model of care, the academic medical center (AMC) tripartite mission needs to be reworked into a new framework that prioritizes management of populations, integration, adaptability, and rapid learning. To complete this change, AMCs will have to undergo the hard work of culture change, which will be facilitated by restructuring governance and organizational structures to fund and champion the population health view. Care coordination and fund health information technology enhancements will be needed to support this work.

PRIMARY CARE:
CLINICS IN OFFICE PRACTICE

SERIES OF RELATED INTEREST

Medical Clinics (http://www.medical.theclinics.com)
Physician Assistant Clinics (http://www.physicianassistant.theclinics.com)

THE CLINICS ARE AVAILABLE ONLINE!
Access your subscription at:
www.theclinics.com

Foreword

Education to Practice, Patients, and Populations

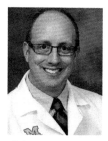

Joel J. Heidelbaugh, MD, FAAFP, FACG
Consulting Editor

Five years ago, a random hallway conversation outside our hospital cafeteria presented an exciting opportunity: would I have an interest in playing a role in developing a new paradigm for our medical school curriculum? The aim would be to create a professional development branch during the third and fourth years of medical school that would allow students to concentrate on elements of medical practice across specialty domains. Recognizing the direction that medicine is heading, a focus on how well we impact the prevention and outcomes of our patients, practices, and populations, I signed up immediately! Thus, the Patients and Populations Branch was born. Today, students who plan to match in both primary care and subspecialty fields incorporate clinical practice, capstone research projects, travel to other academic institutions and abroad, and self-created patient panels within longitudinal clinics to learn provisions of population-based health care.

Over the years, I've heard a lot of people (doctors, administrators, patients) attempt to define and understand what population health is and what it means to them. Years ago, the Institute for Healthcare Improvement developed the Triple Aim concept, highlighting the importance of a balance across managing the health of populations, cost-effective health care, and improving the experience of care. Years later, we still struggle to contain costs, meet patient access and quality metrics, and adequately close the gap on health care disparities. Yet, efforts in both undergraduate medical education and continuing medical education provide expert lectures and materials for us to gain skills and perspectives.

Students across all health professions strive for the ability to learn patient care outside of the limitations of textbooks and wards, incorporating advocacy and public policy, and working toward a creation of new models of health care. Health care providers at all stages of their careers contemplate the impact of change in care delivery and how to provide a better degree of care while minimizing risk of burnout and

Prim Care Clin Office Pract 46 (2019) xiii–xiv
https://doi.org/10.1016/j.pop.2019.09.002
0095-4543/19/© 2019 Published by Elsevier Inc.

maintaining passion for primary care medicine. This issue of *Primary Care: Clinics in Office Practice* highlights well-crafted articles defining population health, preventive medicine, lean thinking, value-based care, viable business models, and strategies for patient engagement across communities and populations. The organization of this issue lends itself on the highest level toward practical application and advancement of medical education on all levels.

I would like to thank Drs Sangvai and Viera, as well as their dedicated and talented article authors, for creating the framework for an innovative and exciting issue of *Primary Care: Clinics in Office Practice* that does an incredible job of presenting both basic and advanced levels of knowledge on population health topics. The perspectives presented herein offer a blueprint for us to better view populations of the patients we serve, always pushing forward to improve health care on a broader level.

Joel J. Heidelbaugh, MD, FAAFP, FACG
Departments of Family Medicine and Urology
University of Michigan Medical School
Ann Arbor, MI 48103, USA

Ypsilanti Health Center
200 Arnet, Suite 200
Ypsilanti, MI 48198, USA

E-mail address:
jheidel@umich.edu

Preface

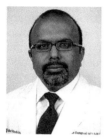
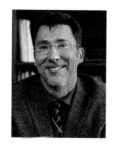

Devdutta G. Sangvai, MD, MBA   Anthony J. Viera, MD, MPH
Editors

We are pleased to bring to you this issue of *Primary Care: Clinics in Office Practice* focused on population health. "Population health" means different things to different people, and while there may be subtle differences in how the term is applied, the tenets of improving health of a population by engaging stakeholders and applying best practices across a spectrum of disciplines are understood by all. Together, the articles in this issue provide a comprehensive understanding of population health. At the same time, each article is designed to engage the reader in a specific element of population health.

Silberberg, Martinez-Bianchi, and Lyn take us through thinking about population health in the broad sense. They use the definition: "the health outcomes of a group of individuals, including the distribution of such outcomes within the group." Of course, we cannot assess the health outcomes of any group without some way to measure health. Coles, Curtis, and Boulware discuss the process of defining metrics that facilitate the documentation of health status. Metrics help measure performance and allow us to decide where to invest resources in efforts to improve population health.

Population health and public health are often confused, and approaches to improve population health include many strategies important to public health, such as "prevention." Marcotte and Dugdale provide a perspective that exemplifies prevention as an important component of population health. Such strategies include the interventions we deliver in clinical settings, such as screening tests, immunizations, preventive medications, and individual counseling. We now have evidence for many effective preventive interventions that can improve population health. However, they can only work if we deliver them to people at the population level. The tools of quality improvement, discussed in the article by Ratner and Pignone, help health care systems assess and address gaps in care delivery. Complementing the tools of quality improvement are ways of managing clinical efforts in the most efficient manner, like the Lean approach described in the article by Anderson, Marstiller, and Shah. Fields and Gandhi highlight the data and analytic, care management, engagement tools, and workflows necessary to be successful in population health management.

https://doi.org/10.1016/j.pop.2019.09.001
0095-4543/19/© 2019 Published by Elsevier Inc.

In all of our efforts to improve health by working with patients, it is vital to remember that the patient is the most important player. Patient engagement, as discussed in the article by Murali and Deao, must be at the heart of our clinical strategies for improving health. Patient-centered care is also the guiding principle of primary care clinic transformation, described in the article by Sawin and O'Connor. Transformed primary care will have a sharp focus on the patient experience of care and will organize services to empower and engage patients to improve their health.

Providing patient-engaged care is ultimately only a part of the full picture of improving population health. To really make a difference in communities, the social determinants of health must be considered, as we read in the article by Houlihan and Leffler. That is why policies are so important and can be the most powerful levers to improve population health as we read in the article by Zolotor and Yorkery. Improving health of communities also requires engagement from stakeholders with whom clinical systems can partner, as discussed in the article by Silberberg and Martinez-Bianchi. Shock further emphasizes this point and outlines how true population health management cannot be realized by entities acting alone nor by solely delivering high-quality care at lower costs. Successful models must also engage partners across their communities to address community culture as well as the broader social determinants of health.

The Triple Aim guides the health care community to think about better care, better health, and better value. Gupta makes the case for value-based care and discusses how key stakeholders, including policy-makers, health systems, patients, and employers, understand how these components of health care value are defined, interlink, and provide opportunities for improvement. Health care reform has been a catalyst for population health, and Wasfy and Ferris make the case that although the pace and details of such payment reforms are uncertain, the underlying structural economic challenges make a transition to some sort of value-based care inevitable. Academic medical centers (AMCs) have unique challenges when it comes to modifying their delivery model to be successful in population health. Conway and Berkowitz outline how AMCs will have to undergo the hard work of culture change—facilitated by restructuring governance and organizational structures to fund and champion population health.

The authors in this issue did an excellent job not only of assembling key ideas but also of providing practical advice or applications. We hope you enjoy and learn from what we believe to be an outstanding and enduring issue of *Primary Care: Clinics in Office Practice*.

Devdutta G. Sangvai, MD, MBA
Department of Family Medicine and Community Health
Duke University
718 Rutherford Street
Durham, NC 27705, USA

Anthony J. Viera, MD, MPH
Department of Family Medicine and Community Health
Duke University
2200 West Main Street, Suite 400
Durham, NC 27705, USA

E-mail addresses:
devdutta.sangvai@duke.edu (D.G. Sangvai)
anthony.viera@duke.edu (A.J. Viera)

What Is Population Health?

Mina Silberberg, PhD[a],*, Viviana Martinez-Bianchi, MD[b],
Michelle J. Lyn, MBA, MHA[c]

KEYWORDS

- Population health • Determinants of health • Practice change
- Health care financing and delivery

KEY POINTS

- There is a call for primary care to engage in population health, but the term is used in diverse ways.
- This article uses the following definition of population health: the health outcomes of a group of individuals, including the distribution of such outcomes within the group.
- Effective population health improvement requires attention to social and environmental, as well as medical, determinants of health. The population health lens can be used at the individual, practice, institutional, and community levels.
- The need for primary care to engage in population health stems from the importance of social and environmental health determinants, the nature of primary care, and contextual changes.
- Population health improvement is promoted by aligned leadership; skills in critical thinking, leadership/teamwork, quality improvement, advocacy, and stakeholder engagement; new financial models; data sharing; supports for practice change; and political will.

WHAT IS POPULATION HEALTH?

A call for US primary care providers (PCPs) to engage in population health is coming from a variety of quarters. An Institute of Medicine report[1] expounds the need for the integration of public health and primary care; that is, "the linkage of programs and activities to promote overall efficiency and effectiveness and achieve gains in population health."[1] The American Academy of Family Physicians[2] encourages its members to understand and engage with these efforts and "urges all national, state, federal, and private

Disclosure: The authors have nothing to disclose.
[a] Duke Division of Community Health, Department of Family Medicine and Community Health, Duke Council on Race and Ethnicity, Duke University, DUMC 104652, Durham, NC 27710, USA;
[b] Duke Department of Family Medicine and Community Health, Duke University, DUMC 3886, 2100 Erwin Road, Durham, NC 27710, USA; [c] Division of Community Health, Department of Family Medicine and Community Health, Duke University, DUMC 104425, Durham, NC 27710, USA
* Corresponding author.
E-mail address: Mina.silberberg@duke.edu
twitter: @vivimbmd (V.M.-B.)

Prim Care Clin Office Pract 46 (2019) 475–484
https://doi.org/10.1016/j.pop.2019.07.001
0095-4543/19/© 2019 Elsevier Inc. All rights reserved.

sector institutions to partner with primary care and public health partners to ensure a more integrated delivery system is provided to improve population health."[2] The American Association of Pediatrics Task Force on Practice Change is promoting use of a population health approach to practice transformation,[3] and the American College of Physicians has called for strengthening the country's public health infrastructure and for collaboration between public health and primary care to promote population health.[4]

Despite this common call to embrace population health, there is variation in how the term is used.[5] The most well-known definition, and the one espoused by the authors, is that of David Kindig and Greg Stoddart,[6] who define population health as "the health outcomes of a group of individuals, including the distribution of such outcomes within the group." They delineate population health as including "health outcomes, patterns of health determinants, and policies and interventions that link these two (**Box 1**)."[6] Population health, then, is the health of populations defined by a variety of factors, such as clinical practice, geographic location, disease status, or social characteristics. Understanding and addressing population health requires identifying the best place to intervene from among the many determinants of a population's health, from the genetic to the social. As shown in **Fig. 1** (the County Health Rankings Model), experts now agree that social and environmental conditions play a larger role in shaping the health of populations than do the biological factors and clinical care that are traditionally associated with health improvement.[7] An effective population-based approach to health therefore requires attention to these social and environmental factors.

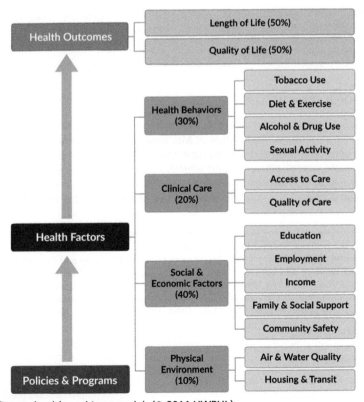

Fig. 1. County health rankings model. (© 2014 UWPHI.)

> **Box 1**
> **Definition of population health**
>
> "Population health is a relatively new term that has not yet been precisely defined… We pro-
> pose that the definition be 'the health outcomes of a group of individuals, including the dis-
> tribution of such outcomes within the group,' and we argue that the field of population
> health includes health outcomes, patterns of health determinants, and policies and interven-
> tions that link these two."[6]

Despite widespread acceptance of Kindig and Stoddart's[6] definition of population health, health professionals on the ground use the term in disparate ways. As argued by Josh Sharfstein[8] in "The Strange Journey of Population Health," the goal of population health researchers in the first part of the millennium was to broaden the discussion of health policy in the United States beyond the biomedical paradigm and to encourage exploration of social determinants of health and health inequality in society as a whole.[8] Insurers and health care providers now use the term to include anything that improves health outcomes, even, he notes, "surgical device management." Sharfstein[8] comments:

It obviously is good news that many in the health care system are now using a term to express their interest in improving the health of those they are serving. It is especially promising that medical students are learning about actions that can help improve the health of groups of patients at a time. But something is lost when the term "population health" is used predominantly by those whose vision may be limited to the group of people they know, see, and track. Poor health is found— indeed, is more likely to be found—among those without a medical home, those shuffling between periods of no health insurance and periods of temporary coverage, and those facing financial, linguistic, and other barriers to care. Initiatives by insurance carriers and clinicians may miss these groups entirely… A bold strategy to improve health must go beyond the usual recommended prevention, clinical quality, data integration, and care coordination efforts. It must extend past what a clinic or insurer can do on its own. It must incorporate social and policy initiatives to improve health, and it must define success or failure by not only those served but also those left behind.

In line with Sharfstein's[8] argument, the authors of this article encourage an approach to population health that incorporates the range of actions that can improve the health of populations but that never loses sight of the profound effect of social and environmental conditions in determining health outcomes. We echo the Institute for Healthcare Improvement, which distinguishes between population medicine ("the design, delivery, coordination, and payment of high-quality health care services to manage the Triple Aim [improved health, improved experience of care and reduced costs[9]] for a population using the best resources we have available to us within the health care system"[10]) and the broader concept of population health, which requires sustainable pragmatic efforts to improve health and health equity through engagement of health care delivery systems and multiple societal stakeholders to address the full range of health determinants.

Arguably, the concept of primary care involvement in population health is not new. Hollander-Rodriguez and DeVoe,[5] along with others, note the synchronicity of calls for primary care to embrace population health with the concept of community-oriented primary care popularized in the 1960s. They note that the 1967 Folsom Report, developed by the National Commission on Community Health Services and sponsored by the American Public Health Association and the National Health Council, "urged primary care physicians to address community health needs by partnering with public health systems and others to create communities of solution that cross jurisdictional lines."[11(p660)]

What PCPs do every day is designed to improve the health of their patients. However, taking a population health perspective can lead providers to think differently about health problems and solutions, and to use their time and resources in very different ways than when they consider the needs of patients 1 at a time.

WHY PRIMARY CARE SHOULD BE INVOLVED IN POPULATION HEALTH

There are several arguments as to why PCPs should be involved with population health. The first has to do with the importance of the social and built environment in shaping health outcomes. PCPs and the patients with whom they work experience the effects of social determinants of health on a daily basis, whether they are aware of it or not.[12] For example, PCPs regularly encounter patients who are unable to afford their prescriptions or patients with asthmatic events triggered by allergens in their homes. Similarly, despite new knowledge regarding nutrition and physical activity, public health professionals are likely to see a growing rate of obesity in their community when residents lack access to healthy foods and safe places to exercise or are overwhelmed by the stresses of their daily lives.[13,14] Put simply, social determinants often confound the efforts of primary care to improve their patients' health. Despite the great gains in knowledge surrounding the science and methods of medicine and prevention, unhealthy environments and social inequalities result in unhealthy lifestyles, deficiencies in medical care and self-management, and health disparities. To make a significant change in population health, primary care professionals will have to collaborate with each other and with other sectors of society to address social and environmental determinants.

Another argument for the involvement of primary care in population health comes from the very conceptualization of primary care. In 1978, in Alma-Ata (in the then Soviet Republic), health experts and world leaders committed to health for all and noted that primary health care:

> Reflects and evolves from the economic conditions and sociocultural and political characteristics of the country and its communities and is based on the application of the relevant results of social, biomedical and health services research and public health experience; and addresses the main health problems in the community, providing promotive, preventive, curative and rehabilitative services accordingly.[15]

The declaration also promoted multisector partnerships to improve health, stating that primary health care involves, in addition to the health sector, all related sectors and aspects of national and community development (agriculture, animal husbandry, food, industry, education, housing, public works, communications, and other sectors) and demands the coordinated efforts of all those sectors. The declaration endorses "maximum community and individual self-reliance and participation in the planning, organization, operation and control of primary health care, making fullest use of local, national and other available resources; and to this end develops through appropriate education the ability of communities." The Global Conference on Primary Health Care in Astana, Kazakhstan, in October of 2018, hosted by the World Health Organization, the United Nations Children's Fund (UNICEF), and the government of Kazakhstan, renewed a global governmental commitment to the critical role of primary health as an indispensable cornerstone to the development goals signed on by all member countries of the United Nations.[16] Population health, then, is arguably integral to primary care and requires looking beyond the individual to the family and community and moving beyond patients seen in the office to the geographic definition of population health used by public health.

In addition, new models of health care delivery and financing are creating incentives for primary care to engage in population health improvement. The Medicare Access and Children's Health Insurance Program Reauthorization Act (MACRA), passed in 2015, represents a particularly important sea change, moving Medicare to a Quality Payment Program in which provider reimbursement is tied to performance metrics designed to incentivize care quality, improve outcomes, and reduce costs across patient panels. The Affordable Care Act incentivizes providers to partner with other sectors to improve population health and reduce health care use. Accountable care organizations, which bring together groups of health care providers to coordinate health care and ancillary services represent one model of health care delivery developed in response to such shifts in financial incentives.

HOW DO PRIMARY CARE PROVIDERS ENGAGE IN POPULATION HEALTH?

Engaging in population health requires providers to follow the basic cycle of assessment, action, and reassessment that they know from individual patient care and continuous quality improvement (QI), but at the level of the population. The process begins with reviewing data to understand a population's health and health needs; for example, identifying poor health outcomes or subgroup health inequities (eg, by age, race/ethnicity, gender, or socioeconomic status) for a clinic's patient panel or catchment area, or comparing data across populations to identify areas of strength and opportunities to improve health. Data are also used to identify the causes of poor health and opportunities for improvement. The assessment process is followed by action to make a positive impact in areas where need is found. Action is followed by reassessment to determine the impact of interventions and determine the next steps.

The population health lens can be used to support action at 4 levels: individual, practice, institutional, and community.[a] For example, a growing number of primary care clinics now employ social workers to whom PCPs can refer individual patients in need of assistance with obtaining food or finding housing. Manchanda,[17] in his TED book, *The Upstream Doctors*, argues that doctors should be assessed in part by the extent to which their care plans take into account an individual patient's social and economic conditions. Similarly, the Health Leads program encourages providers to "prescribe" basic resources, such as food, to individual patients and trains college students to work with patients to connect them with those resources.[18]

Integrating the population health perspective into individual-level patient care is a natural fit with the daily routine, skill set, and comfort zone of providers. However, true population health interventions require going beyond working with individuals, which can be done at the level of a clinical practice, for example, by marking a walking trail on clinic grounds for the use of employees or training providers on unconscious bias or cultural competence. Individual practices operating within a larger institutional setting (eg, an academic medical center) can bring the population health perspective

---

[a] The authors have drawn here on the work of Gottlieb and colleagues,[26] who suggest that PCPs can address social determinants of health on 3 different levels: individual, institutional, and community. We have broken the institutional level into the individual practice and the larger institution with which it might be affiliated, and have expanded the schema beyond social determinants to population health in general.

to decisions and actions of the institution, ranging from replication of successful practice transformation initiatives to adoption of a living wage policy or provision of healthy foods in the hospital cafeteria.

In addition, PCPs can act at the community level (local, state, or national): for example, collaborating with others to identify and address substandard housing that is affecting patient health or advocating for new recreational facilities in communities that have been identified as having a high prevalence of disease or disease risk factors. The greatest gains in population health come when care for individuals is combined with policy change. For example, public sector regulations that prohibited smoking in workplaces and designated public areas were able to reduce odds of smoking by 15% among youth and young adults.[19]

WHAT DOES IT TAKE FOR PRIMARY CARE PROVIDERS TO ENGAGE IN POPULATION HEALTH?

PCPs have several assets for engaging in population health. Patient data can be used to identify patterns of health outcomes that indicate the need to explore social determinants (eg, a pattern of uncontrolled pediatric asthma in one area of town). The stories of individual patients are powerful tools for increasing the visibility of an issue. PCPs can leverage the respect afforded their profession and their expertise about health and illness to increase the awareness of policymakers and the general public about the impact of social conditions on health. They can also leverage their resources as members of the professional class; their access to decision makers, colleagues, and patients; and their role as gatekeepers of health care resources. In one example, in the 1960s, the health council of the Tufts-Delta Health Center in Mound Bayou, Mississippi, helped end discriminatory banking practices by promising local banks that the council's funding would be deposited with the first bank that opened a branch in a black neighborhood and engaged in fair employment and mortgage loan practices.[20]

Internal Factors

As shown in **Table 1**, several factors internal to the clinical practice and health system play a significant role in the capacity of primary care practices to leverage the assets just described and engage effectively in population health improvement.

Table 1
Internal factors facilitating primary clinic involvement in population health

Factor	Examples
Leadership and team skills	Working with interdisciplinary or multisectoral teams, leading change
Critical thinking	Identifying possible root causes of poor health, analyzing or reviewing qualitative and quantitative data to assess and reassess population health
Quality improvement techniques	Using the plan-do-study-act cycle for practice transformation or community change
Advocacy skills	Speaking to legislators, using data on health disparities to support legislative change
Community engagement	Creating referral networks, bringing together multisectoral expertise, advocating for change with others

Leadership and team skills
In order to address population health, PCPs almost always work in teams, sometimes (but not always) in leadership positions. They need to be able to collaborate with diverse groups, support and manage change, communicate effectively, understand roles and responsibilities, and organize and coordinate efforts.

Aligned leadership
In order for primary care practices and delivery systems to participate effectively in population health efforts, leadership must be aligned around both goals and approach. Obtaining data on populations from the electronic medical record, developing care teams able to engage with the community and meet community needs, and creating payment and work time models to support population health work require alignment among executive leadership, medical directors, and leaders from human resources, information technology, and research.

Critical thinking
In order to address population health, clinicians and practice personnel must be able to think critically about the strengths and assets of their clinic, the population with which they are working, and population health interventions. In particular, they must be able to use qualitative and quantitative data to identify population health needs, find possible solutions, and assess their outcomes. For example, they might use data to assess the health status of a population; review HEDIS (Healthcare Effectiveness Data and Information Set) metrics; explore social and behavioral domains; analyze health disparities by ethnicity, gender, sexual orientation, or age; or compare practice data with community and neighborhood indicators.[21]

Quality improvement
QI techniques and skills are useful for efforts to improve population health, whether inside a clinic or, combined with engagement with other sectors, in the larger community. QI projects use iterative rapid cycles of planning, doing, studying, and assessing to try out different approaches to implementing interventions that can improve health.

Advocacy
Advocacy entails engaging legislative decision makers, business, and media to shape public policy to improve population health. Examples may be ensuring access to health care, protecting funding for social services, or advocating reforms to educational systems or community development.

Stakeholder engagement
The efforts of PCPs to improve population health will be amplified through collaboration with other sectors of society. Even identifying the challenges facing 1 individual (eg, poverty, lack of housing, untreated mental health problems) and connecting that person to resources will be greatly facilitated by combining the access of clinics with the resources of public health and social services agencies. Going beyond the individual to address health at the population level requires change in economic structures, political systems, cultural systems, social institutions, and/or social policies. Promoting this kind of change requires the expertise and assets of individuals and organizations from a variety of sectors, such as medicine, public health, housing, education, community organizing, and government.

External Factors

In addition to the internal characteristics of medical practices, external factors play a significant role in promoting or impeding effective population health efforts. This article discusses 4 key factors: health care financing, data sharing, support for practice change, and political will (**Table 2**).

Health care financing

It has long been understood that health care financing plays a crucial role in shaping population health efforts (or lack thereof).[22] The traditional fee-for-service payment system encourages providers to provide more services and procedures to those who can pay for them, not to improve health for populations. Capitation, bundled payments, or other ways of tying payment to individuals or episodes of health create incentives for less use of expensive services, but do not intrinsically create incentives for health improvement. Some cost-cutting measures (eg, effective use of preventive services) can both improve health and save money over the long-term, whereas others only save money. However, much of the cost saving associated with prevention occurs over the long-term, when it is likely that patients will have moved on to new payers and providers, decreasing the incentive for current payers and providers to invest in prevention. Moreover, alternatives to fee for service can promote cost shifting from one clinical setting to another, one patient group to another, or one payer to another, rather than encouraging a systemic approach to improving health and saving money.

As noted earlier, experimentation is taking place with more sophisticated approaches to health care financing that integrate new forms of payment with mechanisms for population health measurement, new delivery models, and even multisectoral collaboration to address social and environmental determinants of health. For example, the Centers for Medicare & Medicaid Services is testing whether an accountable health communities model of systematically identifying and addressing the health-related social needs of Medicare and Medicaid beneficiaries through screening, referral, and community navigation services can improve health while reducing health care costs.[23] The primary idea behind these new financing experiments is that the dollars should pay for value, in the form of improved population health, rather than for services. Of course, the impact of these experiments will be limited if the population whose health they address is limited to specific groups of covered lives.

Data sharing

Another factor that can facilitate population health improvement is the sharing of data to identify health problems and root causes, plan potential solutions, and evaluate

---

Table 2
External factors facilitating primary clinic involvement in population health

Factor	Examples
Health care financing	Fee for service promotes services and procedures, not population health. Capitation can create incentives for less use of expensive services, but not always health improvement. New approaches combine new payment models with new delivery models
Data sharing	Data from health care, public health, and other sectors can be combined to identify health problems and root causes, plan potential solutions, and evaluate their results
Support for practice change	Technical assistance, ramp-up time, flexibility
Political will	Willingness to support change in the health care system, the policies that govern it, its institutional settings, and social and environmental conditions

their results.[1] For example, through the Primary Care Information Project, the New York City Department of Mental Health and Hygiene integrates electronic health record data from clinical sites into a population health registry that can be used to assess health outcomes, including disparities, across the city.[24] However, data sharing has several challenges, including privacy concerns and regulatory barriers, incompatible data systems, competing interests, and lack of buy-in. Even when data are shared, the effectiveness of this sharing can be limited by the quality and timeliness of the data. Approaches to addressing the challenges of data sharing are being studied and disseminated.[25]

Support for practice change

Ironically, the call for health care systems change can be an impediment to its own fulfillment. Rapid, uncertain, or dramatic external change can be generative or destructive (or both) in the life of an organization. Practice transformation to improve population health requires not only that primary care practices be ready to make needed changes (a goal that it is hoped will be in part supported by this issue of *Primary Care*) but that external conditions provide them with the technical assistance, ramp-up time, and flexibility to do so.

Political will

All 3 of the external factors discussed so far (financing, data sharing, and support for practice change) show the importance of a fourth factor: political will. The conditions for population health improvement, and the effective participation of primary care in this endeavor, will not be met without the willingness of both public and private decision makers to support change in the health care system, the policies that govern it, its institutional settings, and the social and environmental conditions that are so fundamental to health. There is a need, therefore, for PCPs to partner with others to advocate for and effect change in a variety of realms and at multiple levels of society.

REFERENCES

1. IOM. Primary care and public health: exploring integration to improve population health. Washington, DC: The National Academies Press; 2012.
2. American Academy of Family Physicians. Integration of primary care and public health 2015.
3. Perrin JM, Edwards AR. AAP task force adding to resources on pediatric practice change. AAP News 2016. Available at: http://www.aappublications.org/news/2016/06/02/PracticeChange060216. Accessed December 20, 2018.
4. ACP. Strengthening the public health infrastructure. Philadelphia: American College of Physicians; 2012.
5. Hollander-Rodriguez J, DeVoe JE. Family medicine's task in population health: defining it and owning it. Fam Med 2018;50(9):659–61.
6. Kindig D, Stoddart G. What is population health? Am J Public Health 2003;93(3): 380–3.
7. University of Wisconsin Population Health Institute. County health rankings model 2014.
8. Sharfstein J. The strange journey of population health. Milbank Mem Fund Q 2014;92(4):640–3.
9. Berwick DM, Nolan TW, Whittington J. The triple aim: care, health, and cost. Health Aff (Millwood) 2008;27(3):759–69.
10. Lewis N. Populations, population health, and the evolution of population management: making sense of the terminology in US health care today. Improvement IfH;

2014. Available at: http://www.ihi.org/communities/blogs/population-health-population-management-terminology-in-us-health-care.

11. NCCHS. Health is a community affair—report of the National Commission on Community Health Services (NCCHS). Cambridge, MA: Harvard University Press; 1967.

12. Bond ANYT. Can you afford your medicine? Doctors don't ask. Times NY 2014.

13. Acevedo-Garcia D, Osypuk TL, McArdle N, et al. Toward a policy-relevant analysis of geographic and racial/ethnic disparities child health. Health Affairs 2008; 27(2):321–33.

14. Diez Roux AV. Investigating neighborhood and area effects on health. AJPH 2001;91:1783–9.

15. Declaration of Alma-Ata. Paper presented at: International Conference on Primary Health Care; September 6–12, 1978; Alma-Ata, USSR.

16. Declaration of Astana. Paper presented at: Global Conference on Primary Health Care. Astana, Kazakhstan, October 25–26, 2018.

17. Manchanda R. The upstream doctors: medical innovators track sickness to its source. TED Books; 2013.

18. Health Leads. Available at: https://healthleadsusa.org/. Accessed December 21, 2018.

19. Levy DT, Tam J, Kuo C, et al. The impact of implementing tobacco control policies: the 2017 Tobacco Control Policy Scorecard. J Public Health Manag Pract 2018;24(5):448–57.

20. Geiger H. Community-oriented primary care: a path to community development. Am J Public Health 2002;92(11):1713–6.

21. NAS. A framework for educating health professionals to address the social determinants of health. Washington, DC: The National Academies Press; 2016.

22. Kindig D. Purchasing population health: aligning financial incentives to improve health outcomes. Health Serv Res 1998;33(2):223–42.

23. Accountable health communities model. Available at: https://innovation.cms.gov/initiatives/ahcm/. Accessed December 21, 2018.

24. Primary care information project. Available at: https://www1.nyc.gov/site/doh/providers/resources/primary-care-information-project.page. Accessed December 21, 2018.

25. Eckart P. Improving health through data sharing: what have we learned? Practical Playbook Blog 2017;2018.

26. Gottlieb L, Sandel M, Adler NE. Collecting and applying data on social determinants of health in health care settings. JAMA Intern Med 2013;173(11):1017–20.

Measuring Health

Theresa M. Coles, PhD[a],*, Lesley H. Curtis, PhD[a,b,c],
L. Ebony Boulware, MD[a,c,d,1]

KEYWORDS

- Population health • Health measurement • Primary care • Metric

KEY POINTS

- Population health addresses the health status of populations. In order to improve population health, one must define metrics that facilitate the documentation of health needs and progress.
- Population health metrics provide information on the health and distribution of health outcomes within population subgroups.
- Strong population health metrics are valid, consistent, feasible to collect, easily interpretable, evaluated longitudinally, and actionable.

INTRODUCTION

Primary care clinicians provide health care for patients experiencing the full spectrum of health and illness, ranging from healthy patients seeking preventive care to patients with complex comorbidities. By managing the full spectrum of health concerns for their patients, primary care clinicians often represent a critical point of contact within health care for preventive and new health concerns, and they provide coordinated and continuous care and support for patients throughout their lives.[1] The breadth of health status among patients seen in primary care was recently quantified in a study conducted within fee-for-service health care networks. Family physicians used almost 10 times the number of International Statistical Classification of Diseases (ICD) diagnosis codes compared with other specialty physicians.[2] Thus, compared with

Disclosure Statement: L.H. Curtis discloses the following commercial funding relationships: Novartis, GlaxoSmithKline, Boston Scientific, St. Jude. All of L.H. Curtis' research contracts are with Duke or DCRI; no consulting or personal compensation has been provided by any commercial funding. T.M. Coles discloses the following commercial funding relationship: Regenxbio. L.E. Boulware does not have commercial funding relationships to disclose.
[a] Department of Population Health Sciences, Duke University, 215 Morris Street, Durham, NC 27701, USA; [b] Duke Clinical Research Institute, Duke University, Durham, NC, USA; [c] Department of Medicine, Duke University, Durham, NC, USA; [d] Department of Community and Family Medicine, Duke University, Durham, NC, USA
[1] Present address: 411 West Chapel Hill Street, Suite 500, Durham, NC 27701.
* Corresponding author. 215 Morris St, Durham, NC 27701.
E-mail address: Theresa.Coles@Duke.edu

Prim Care Clin Office Pract 46 (2019) 485–491
https://doi.org/10.1016/j.pop.2019.07.002
0095-4543/19/© 2019 Elsevier Inc. All rights reserved.

specialty clinicians, primary care clinicians are uniquely poised to measure and address the health of many diverse patient populations.

It has long been intuited that measuring health is the first step in understanding health, and understanding health is the first step in improving health. Population health activities ascertain and address the health status of aggregate populations (ie, groups of patients), including the distribution of population health outcomes.[3] Because populations are comprised of individuals, an initial step required to evaluate distributions of health at a population level is the measurement of indicators of health for individual patients. Once these measures are performed, they can be aggregated to develop insights about groups of patients representing specific populations of interest. Thus, measurement of health among individuals is integral to understanding the health of populations.

With burgeoning electronic health records, primary care clinicians are now able to develop their own metrics to measure the health of individual patients and to better understand and characterize the aggregate health of populations (ie, patient panels) for whom they provide care. Health systems or clinical practices may also choose their own metrics to measure population health. Quality measures (eg, Healthcare Effectiveness Data and Information Set [HEDIS] and Physician Quality Reporting System [PQRS]) are the most common metrics used in practice, because they are tied to reimbursement or payment through insurance. Insurance groups choose which metrics they will use to define quality and then reimburse or pay providers who achieve those metrics. Although quality measurement intends to provide a framework for measuring the quality of care, metrics are presented as simple numbers and provide only a limited view of population health. Population health measurement will become increasingly relevant as Medicare payment initiatives shift from fee-for-service to clinicians being accountable for the health of their population with financial implications. Value-based initiatives focus on outcomes, which will be addressed with population-level metrics.

For all population metrics, there are important considerations regarding the strengths and limitations of each measure, and how metrics can be used to drive action. This article considers examples of population-level metrics employed in primary care practices, the characteristics of measures, and their potential use to spur action to improve the health of populations in primary care.

CHARACTERISTICS OF POPULATION HEALTH MEASURES

All population health metrics have characteristics that influence the extent to which they are useful, informative, and actionable. These characteristics include their validity, consistency, feasibility, interpretability, and assessment time frame (**Table 1**).

Table 1 Characteristics of population health metrics that influence usefulness	
Characteristics of Population Health Metrics	**Description**
Valid	Metrics that measure what is intended to be measured
Consistent	Metrics that are well-defined and can be measured the same way across practices or populations
Feasible	Metrics that are measured in practical ways that do not place undue burden on patients, clinicians, or systems
Interpretable	Metrics that stakeholders can understand in order to take action
Longitudinal	Metrics that track health over time to provide insight into populations' health improvements or declines

Valid Metrics: Measuring What Is Intended to Be Measured

A valid population health metric must specifically measure a condition of interest and not a related condition. For example, the patient-reported outcome (PRO) Patient Health Questionnaire (PHQ-9)[4] was developed to measure symptoms of depression, but this measure does not assess related conditions such as anxiety, and it does not provide information on important contextual concerns such as social support. Although tools such as the PHQ-9 are often administered to individual patients for diagnostic purposes, they can also be administered to multiple patients in a clinic for surveillance purposes, providing information on groups of patients. Scores from these measures can be aggregated, and their distributions (eg, mean, median, range) can be reviewed. Score distributions can be used to understand the prevalence of conditions at a single point in time or changes in scores over longer periods of time to determine if depressive symptoms are improving or worsening in the clinic's population. Information from this type of assessment can be used to inform administrative or clinical actions. For instance, high rates of depressive symptoms among clinic patients might lead primary care physicians to implement changes in clinic practice such as enhanced referrals to mental health professionals.

It is important to distinguish between metrics that evaluate the process of care delivery and those that evaluate health. Specifically, some quality metrics evaluate the proportion of encounters in which a PRO measure has been administered to patients[5] rather than the distribution of PRO scores collected from the patients. Metrics focused on administration of PRO measures rather than the distribution of patient scores do not directly evaluate patients' health. Thus, process metrics may not indicate whether patients' health can be improved through action.

Consistent Metrics

Consistent metrics are well-defined and applied in a similar manner across practices or populations. A metric can be valid if one measures what one intends to measure about health, but not consistent if one measures health differently in different situations. For example, one primary care practice could estimate the proportion of individuals in the past year who were vaccinated for influenza and subsequently diagnosed with influenza. Another primary care practice could estimate the proportion of individuals diagnosed with influenza in the past year overall (regardless of vaccination status). Although these metrics are similar, they are not consistent and cannot be used to compare influenza rates across practices, because the proportion of individuals with influenza is calculated with different denominators. For the first practice, the denominator would be the patients vaccinated for influenza, and for the second practice, the denominator is all patients in the practice. Similarly, metrics should be applied consistently within practices over time. If population health metrics change over time, one is unable to compare improvements or worsening in health outcomes from month to month. Consistent use of metrics is becoming particularly important in light of mounting interest in team-based primary care.[6,7] When multiple clinical teams seek to measure health status across their populations and share best practices, they may benefit most when measuring health using consistent, valid metrics that facilitate cross-team comparisons.

Feasible Metrics

Not all aspects of population health can be measured feasibly. For example, the frequency with which patients experience asthma exacerbations at home is an indicator of asthma severity. However, patients presenting to the clinic may not be able to recall asthma exacerbation intensity at home accurately if time has passed since exacerbations, or if at-home administration of questionnaires is not feasible. In addition, patients may not be able to accurately recall the frequency and severity of asthmatic episodes that occur over long periods of time. A more feasible measure of asthma severity could be the dispensing of asthma rescue medications. For instance, HEDIS collects information on dispensing of asthma medications for individuals aged 5 to 85 years,[8] making the availability of this information more feasible than patient self-reported asthma exacerbations at home. Despite this, the dispensing of asthma rescue medications is a distal indicator of actual asthma-related health and may not reflect patients' asthma control. Further, dispensing does not indicate that patients took the medication as intended.

Similarly, it might be possible to measure sleep quality for a small group of patients in the laboratory. However, evaluating sleep quality for all patients in a population via laboratory-based measures is not feasible. Given a small sample of individuals who could feasibly be evaluated via laboratory-based sleep measures, clinicians should note that metrics obtained at a population level based on intensive laboratory measures may be skewed or biased, because they represent only a small proportion of the population who needed or could obtain the sleep laboratory-based metrics. A more feasible approach to measuring sleep quality in a population could be to administer a screening questionnaire in the clinic to identify patient reports of sleep disturbances. For example, the Insomnia Severity Index[9] is a psychometrically evaluated questionnaire that could be administered electronically. Questionnaire scores could be calculated electronically, and predefined thresholds could be used to identify patients in need of support from a psychologist trained in Cognitive Behavioral Therapy for Insomnia (CBT-I). The proportion of patients who exceed a threshold indicating poor sleep could be calculated to indicate the overall sleep health of the clinic's population.

Interpretable Metrics

Metrics must be interpretable to be useful. If information obtained from metrics is unclear, necessary actions to address a potential population health problem are also unclear. For example, because of recent changes in blood pressure classification guidelines,[10,11] many individuals once categorized as exhibiting normal blood pressure have now been reclassified as hypertensive. Depending on a clinic's case mix and the metrics used to describe cardiovascular health within the clinic, the population may appear less healthy simply because of the new guidelines. In this case, primary care clinicians must interpret blood pressure control metrics in the context of the changing blood pressure guidelines in order to understand that changes in measured population health status may be driven by a change in guidelines, not by care in the clinical practice or actual patient health status.

The ability to drill down on (or segment) population data for particular population subgroups is important in interpreting metrics. Evaluating data obtained from subgroups of a population can help primary care clinicians direct resources to groups in most need of intervention to improve practice efficiency and effectiveness.[12] For instance, when measuring depressive symptoms in a primary care population, worsening average depressive symptom scores over time could signal that the overall patient population is experiencing increasingly severe depressive symptoms. Or, drilling down further, worsening scores could be caused by the influx of new patients whose symptoms have not yet been addressed or perhaps new patients who have not yet been referred to a psychologist. These possibilities could be evaluated by comparing the distributions of PHQ-9 scores among specific segments of the overall population: new patients versus existing patients.

Longitudinal Metrics

Some metrics can be most useful when they provide insight on the health of a population over time. For example, if a primary care clinic is seeking to improve the rates of diabetes control in their practice, a metric on the prevalence of poor glucose control (eg, HbA1c) obtained in a population at a single time point may not be very informative. However, tracking the prevalence of poor glucose control in the clinic population over time could allow clinicians to observe improvement or worsening in glucose control over time, and to direct actions to improve care.

Taking Action

Population health metrics best support primary care patients and clinicians when they are actionable. Eidus and colleagues[13] categorized activities to address population health problems as high-leverage or low-leverage activities (**Table 2**). High-leverage activities greatly influence clinical outcomes in the short term and the long term and generally require more effort or resources to implement. For example, if a population health metric showed that half of a clinic population had high blood pressure, a high-leverage approach could include a program to ensure clinic nurses address all patients' adherence to blood pressure medications during their clinic visits. However, this high-leverage intervention might be time consuming for staff, and may be infeasible or unsustainable because of budget and time constraints. By contrast, low-leverage activities are activities that exert less influence on clinical outcomes and may require less effort or resources to implement. For instance, informational pamphlets explaining proper high blood pressure management could be placed in each clinic room. This intervention would be considered a low-leverage activity, because the pamphlets would influence hypertension metrics indirectly.

Ideally, well-selected population health metrics should inform not only whether high- or low-leverage actions should be taken, but also how effective the actions are over time. The choice of using high- or low-leverage activities to address population health should be contextualized within evidence-based considerations for impact, burden, cost, and benefit. It is possible that high-leverage activities, although likely more time consuming and costly, may result in better outcomes and reduced costs overall.[13] Studies may be warranted to evaluate the balance between resources needed and benefits achieved, and which metrics ideally measure outcomes. Further, new metrics may need to be developed to measure the effectiveness of the high- or low-leverage activities.

Table 2 High- and low- leverage activities in primary care		
	High-Leverage Activities	**Low-Leverage Activities**
Definition	• Greatly influence clinical outcomes in short term and long term	• Exert less influence on clinical outcomes
Considerations	• Often require more effort or resources to implement • May be difficult to sustain over time • May be more beneficial or cost-effective	• Often require less effort or resources to implement • May be less beneficial or cost-effective

SUMMARY

Primary care clinicians care for an extremely diverse range of patients, and they therefore have numerous opportunities to measure and act to improve the health of populations. In order to take effective actions to improve the health of their patient populations, primary care clinicians must utilize measures with optimum validity, consistency, feasibility, interpretability, and assessment time frame. The strongest metrics are actionable, supporting the implementation of effective interventions that can lead to improvements in patients' health.

ACKNOWLEDGMENTS

The authors would like to thank Matthew Higgins, Manager of Performance Services, Duke Regional Hospital, for health measurement insights.

REFERENCES

1. Starfield B. Is primary care essential? Lancet 1994;344(8930):1129–33.
2. Cunningham CT, Cai P, Topps D, et al. Mining rich health data from Canadian physician claims: features and face validity. BMC Res Notes 2014;7:682.
3. Centers for Disease Control and Prevention. What is Population Health?. 2018. Available at: https://www.cdc.gov/pophealthtraining/whatis.html. Accessed November 21, 2018.
4. Kroenke K, Spitzer RL, Williams JBW. The PHQ-9 - Validity of a brief depression severity measure. J Gen Intern Med 2001;16(9):606–13.
5. National Committee for Quality Assurance (NCQA). Depression screening and follow-up for adolescents and adults (DSF). 2018. Available at: https://www.ncqa.org/hedis/measures/depression-screening-and-follow-up-for-adolescents-and-adults/. Accessed November 21, 2018.
6. Riverin BD, Li P, Naimi AI, et al. Team-based versus traditional primary care models and short-term outcomes after hospital discharge. CMAJ 2017;189(16):E585–93.
7. Wagner EH, Flinter M, Hsu C, et al. Effective team-based primary care: observations from innovative practices. BMC Fam Pract 2017;18(1):13.
8. National Committee for Quality Assurance (NCQA). Medication management for people with asthma and asthma medication ratio (MMA, AMR). 2018. Available at: https://www.ncqa.org/hedis/measures/medication-management-for-people-with-asthma-and-asthma-medication-ratio/. Accessed November 21, 2018.
9. Gagnon C, Belanger L, Ivers H, Morin CM. Validation of the Insomnia Severity Index in Primary Care. Journal of the American Board of Family Medicine 2013; 26(6):701–10.
10. Whelton PK, Carey RM, Aronow WS, et al. 2017 ACC/AHA/AAPA/ABC/ACPM/AGS/APhA/ASH/ASPC/NMA/PCNA guideline for the prevention, detection, evaluation, and management of high blood pressure in adults: executive summary: a report of the American College of Cardiology/American Heart Association Task Force on Clinical Practice Guidelines. Hypertension 2018;71(6):1269–324.
11. Whelton PK, Carey RM, Aronow WS, et al. 2017 ACC/AHA/AAPA/ABC/ACPM/AGS/APhA/ASH/ASPC/NMA/PCNA guideline for the prevention, detection, evaluation, and management of high blood pressure in adults: a report of the American College of Cardiology/American Heart Association Task Force on Clinical Practice Guidelines. Hypertension 2018;71(6):e13–115.

12. Langton JM, Wong ST, Johnston S, et al. Primary Care performance measurement and reporting at a regional level: could a matrix approach provide actionable information for policy makers and clinicians? Health Policy 2016;12(2): 33–51.
13. Eidus R, Pace WD, Staton EW. Managing patient populations in primary care: points of leverage. J Am Board Fam Med 2012;25(2):238–44.

Prevention as a Population Health Strategy

Leah M. Marcotte, MD[a], David C. Dugdale, MD[b],*

KEYWORDS

- Population health • Preventive health • Community linkages
- Community health workers • Health coaches

KEY POINTS

- Evidence-based prevention strategies promote improved health outcomes on population levels and decrease costs to the health care system.
- Community linkages to promote preventive services are effective, especially in partnership with primary care services.
- Barriers to population-based approaches include the fee-for-service payment model and lack of community-based partners within primary care service areas.

INTRODUCTION

High-value care has increasing traction within health policy and health care delivery systems, with population health outcomes being an important piece of quality of care. Although improving the health of populations is a relatively new concept in most primary care practices, there is substantial experience within public health and community-based programs that can help health care organizations to approach population-based care.

HISTORY OF PREVENTIVE MEDICINE AND POPULATION-BASED APPROACHES

Health care delivery affects only an estimated 10% of health outcomes, whereas behavioral factors account for approximately 40% and social and environmental factors approximately 20%.[1] Therefore, in order to effectively have an impact on population health in primary care settings, behavioral interventions and approaches to social

Disclosure Statement: The authors have nothing to disclose.
[a] Division of General Internal Medicine, Department of Medicine, University of Washington School of Medicine, Suite 355, 1107 Northeast 45th Street, Seattle, WA 98105, USA; [b] Division of General Internal Medicine, Department of Medicine, University of Washington School of Medicine, Suite 355, 1107 Northeast 45th Street, Seattle, WA 98105, USA
* Corresponding author.
E-mail address: dugdaled@uw.edu

and environmental determinants of health should be integrated into preventive medicine approaches.

In his seminal book, Rose[2] explains preventive medicine as managing risk of disease across a population and both risk and disease as spectra affecting individuals to different degrees. Population-based approaches may focus on high-risk populations or average-risk populations. Rose argues that any risk that is distributed across a population (vs limited to a discrete segment of a population) is best approached by focusing on improving average risk. He gives several reasons for this. First, there often are more cases of disease in the average-risk category than in the high-risk population. Second, small improvements on a population level frequently also affect behavior and reduce risk of the extreme or deviant population. In other words, shifting the mean of the distribution curve slightly can substantially affect the tail.

In 2010, Frieden[3] introduced the health impact pyramid, which ranks population-based interventions by effort and impact. In order of highest overall impact and lowest individual effort needed the tiers are as follows: (1) socioeconomic factors (base of pyramid), (2) changing context in order to default to healthy decisions, (3) protective interventions that are long lasting, (4) clinical interventions, and (5) counseling and education (pyramid tip).[3] Primary care delivery typically focuses in clinical interventions and counseling and education—the lowest impact, highest individual-effort population-based interventions. Although primary care may have limited direct leverage to affect the highest-impact interventions in the health impact pyramid, there is opportunity to partner with community-based programs that may be better equipped to address behavioral, social, and environmental determinants of health.

Among clinical preventive interventions, there are varying levels of effectiveness and impact. A 2006 review found that highest-impact, lowest-cost services include discussing aspirin use with high-risk adults, pediatric immunizations, and tobacco screening and brief intervention.[4] The investigators also identified high-ranked services that were underutilized, including colorectal cancer screening, chlamydia screening in young women, and pneumococcal vaccine for adults 65 years old or older.

Several recent studies model potential clinical and financial impacts of preventive services. In 2010, Maciosek and colleagues[5] estimated that delivering 20 evidence-based preventive services to 90% of the United States population would prevent 2 million life-years lost and save $3.7 billion per year compared with baseline services delivered in 2006. In a similar analysis, Farley and colleagues[6] concluded that focused improvement on a small number of preventive services could lead to considerable improvements in mortality. For example, improving hypertension treatment by 10% could prevent 14,000 deaths per year and lowering low-density lipoprotein cholesterol or improving appropriate increased aspirin use could prevent 8000 deaths per year.

POPULATION-BASED APPROACH TO DISEASE PREVENTION

Population-based prevention is a relatively new activity for primary care practices in the United States. Improved health information technology and team-based models of care may enable primary care to expand traditional scope of practice to include population-based management without over-burdening providers. A model that identifies 10 building blocks of high-performing primary care—including data-driven improvement, team-based care, empanelment, and population management also supports population-based approaches to prevention.[7]

Empanelment defines the population for which a primary care provider or practice is accountable. Health information technology tools can capture and display population-level information on quality dashboards customized to an individual provider or practice. Rather than adding to the administrative burden of primary care providers, teams can effectively manage population-based preventive health care. Common tactics include standing orders for cancer screening services, such as mammograms or fecal immunochemical tests (FITs). Medical assistants, health coaches, or health care navigators can identify care gaps and outreach to patients outside of face-to-face visits.

Population-based approaches to prevention can improve preventive service delivery. In a randomized control trial of more than 40,000 patients, an intervention of an introductory letter, followed by a FIT card and reminder letter, created an increased colorectal cancer screening rate: 18.3% compared with 14.5% for usual care.[8] Removing barriers by mailing a FIT card and colorectal cancer screening reminder to a group of Medicaid patients increased screening completion rates to 21.1% in comparison to 12.3% in the control group who received a reminder letter alone.[9]

There are several common barriers to effective population-based management in primary care practices. Most primary care in the United States is delivered predominantly under a fee-for-service payment model, which fails to incentivize non–face-to-face care. That is changing with evolving payer policies; however, existing bonuses for performance metrics often do not cover the additional resources needed to identify patients due for care and subsequent outreach. Although many systems are innovating and there are some emerging best practices, there are still limited experience and guidance on care team structures and training to most effectively do population-based management.

HEALTH COACHING AND DISEASE PREVENTION

The advent of team-based care has increased interest in training staff members to be health coaches for patients in individual or group settings. In the context of chronic illness care, health coaching aims to engage patients with chronic conditions in their care by increasing their "knowledge, skills, and confidence," thus reducing their consequences.[10] In theory, a similar model applies to primary prevention but there are fewer data in this domain (**Box 1**).[11]

Most trials have focused on patients with a specific chronic illness, with benefits shown in type 2 diabetes mellitus (T2D),[12] hypertension,[13] and cardiovascular disease risk factors[14] but not in patients with chronic obstructive pulmonary disease.[15] Health coaching was associated with an increased trust in primary care.[16] A time study of health coaches in 3 federally qualified health centers in San Francisco found that coaches participated in 70% of medical visits, spending a mean of 15 minutes before the visit, primarily on activities that bridged communication between patients and clinicians to improve chronic disease management.[17]

Box 1
Core principles of health coaching

Ask-tell-ask

Closing the loop, or teach back

Know your numbers

Behavior-change action plans

Medication adherence counseling

Data from Goldman ML, Ghorob A, Hessler D, et al. Are low-income peer health coaches able to master and utilize evidence-based health coaching? Ann Fam Med 2015;13(Suppl 1):S36-S41.

A growing approach to health coaching uses digitally connected coaches or virtual communities provided by a vendor paid by an employer or health plan. An example to support chronic illness care, Livongo for Diabetes, uses proprietary technology to connect people with diabetes to certified diabetes educators. Published reports are promising[18,19]; however, scalability, sustainability, and how best to avoid siloing of care remain uncertain.

Many employers offer virtual health coaching and wellness programs for employees as part of their health benefit package. For example, Omada Health, a 16-week program for diabetes prevention in those at increased risk of T2D, is conceptually similar to the Diabetes Prevention Program (DPP) (discussed later). Although published results are promising, long-term impacts and scalability remain uncertain.[20]

Data on the effect of health coaching on disease prevention or risk factor reduction show mixed results. Of 7 primary prevention interventions, 5 were conducted with employees. Four of the 7 interventions showed some improvement in psychological or behavioral variables that might improve health status.[21]

COMMUNITY-CLINICAL LINKAGES

There is good reason to believe that community-clinical linkages can allow for greater dissemination and impact of effective interventions into communities. Porterfield and colleagues[22] identified 49 interventions that linked primary care practices and community agencies, some of which were effective, but concluded that the evidence was insufficient to support the effectiveness of such models. By 2016, the Centers for Disease Control and Prevention (CDC)[23] published a best practice guide to support this work (**Box 2**).

Community Linkages and Diabetes Prevention

Upwards of 28 million Americans have T2D, with another 84 million having prediabetes. In 2017, the cost of diabetes and prediabetes to Americans was $322 billion.[24] Although not all cases of T2D are preventable, effective prevention is available. The DPP tested the effect of metformin or intensive lifestyle modification (goals of at least a 7% weight loss and 150 minutes of physical activity per week) in people at elevated risk of developing T2D.[25] The Diabetes Prevention Program Outcomes Study (DPPOS)[26] examined the long-term effects. These results (**Table 1**) are the basis of subsequent program development.

A modification of the DPP, the group-organized YMCA DPP, aims for a 5% weight loss and 150 minutes per week of exercise, has a group format (10–12 participants), and lasts 16 weeks.[27,28] This reduced the per-participant cost from $1400 in the

---

Box 2

Strategies for planning and implementing community-clinical linkages

L	Learn about community and clinical sectors.
I	Identify and engage key stakeholders from community clinical sectors.
N	Negotiate and agree on goals objectives of the linkage.
K	Know which operational structure to implement.
A	Aim to coordinate and manage the linkage.
G	Grow the linkage with sustainability in mind.
E	Evaluate the linkage.

From Centers for Disease Control and Prevention. Community-clinical linkages for the prevention and control of chronic diseases: A practitioner's guide. Atlanta, GA: Centers for Disease Control and Prevention, U.S. Department of Health and Human Services; 2016.

Table 1 Reduction of type 2 diabetes mellitus incidence by the Diabetes Prevention Program		
Mean Length of Follow-up (y)	Metformin, 850 mg, Twice Daily	Intensive Lifestyle Modification
2.8 (DPP)	31%	58%
10 (DPPOS)	18%	34%

original DPP to $275 to $325, while maintaining effectiveness. The Diabetes Prevention Act of 2009 catalyzed large-scale capacity building for delivering some version of the DPP, often via community agencies. The CDC developed a DPP recognition program and created messaging about this to medical practitioners. In late 2018, in the United States, there were 310 fully recognized programs, 261 with preliminary recognition, and 1220 with pending recognition.[29]

At-risk Medicare beneficiaries who participated in a YMCA DPP realized a $278 per quarter health cost savings driven in part by a decrease in inpatient and emergency department visits of 9 of each per 1000 participants per quarter.[30] These results led the Centers for Medicare & Medicaid Services to cover these programs under specific circumstances, effective April 1, 2018.

Community Linkages and Physical Activity

The "Physical Activity Guidelines for Americans, 2nd edition," highlight the benefits of physical activity on health.[31] The Exercise is Medicine campaign, launched in 2007 enunciated a vision of care that includes universal assessment of activity at medical visits, brief advice, and referral for detailed physical activity counseling.[32] Emphasizing the importance of community linkages, the National Physical Activity Plan[33] recognizes the need for efforts in 9 societal sectors outside of health care organizations (**Box 3**).

The National Physical Activity Plan includes strategies, tactics, and examples of successful programs and has an accompanying implementation guide.[34] For many adults, workplace-based interventions may be particularly convenient.[35] Evidence remains limited, however, and most implementations do not provide a rigorous analysis.

Box 3 Societal sectors of the National Physical Activity Plan
Business and industry
Community recreation, fitness, and parks
Education
Faith-based settings
Health care
Mass media
Public health
Sport
Transportation, land use, and community design
Data from National Physical Activity Plan 2016. Available at: http://www.physicalactivityplan.org/theplan/about.html (accessed November 23, 2018).

A group with a more robust evidence base is elderly people. Beyond the multiple benefits cited for the benefits of physical activity in the general population is the reduction of falls and higher functional status in the elderly.[36] For example, EnhanceFitness, originally created as a partnership between community agencies and Group Health Cooperative in Seattle, Washington, is a low-cost, adaptable, group exercise program for older adults.[37] Almost 20 years later, it remains a program with which clinicians can collaborate.[38]

Community Linkages and Social Isolation

Loneliness and social isolation are an increasingly studied and recognized social determinant of health. Social isolation is an objective concept tied to social interactions, social support, and engagement with others.[39,40] Loneliness reflects the "degree of mismatch between desired and actual social relationships."[39] Social isolation occurs in 17% to 43% of adults 60 years and older in the United States.[41] The prevalence of loneliness among adults age 65 years and older in the United States is 30% to 60%.[40,42]

Loneliness and social isolation have a health impact comparable to smoking, alcohol consumption, physical inactivity, and obesity.[41] Loneliness is associated with functional decline and death in people age 60 and older.[43] Among enrollees in an American Association of Retired Persons (AARP) Medicare Supplement Plan who were eligible for care management services, 28% reported severe loneliness and 27% reported moderate loneliness.[44] Depression; being female; having vision, hearing, and walking/balance problems; having poorer health; and urban location were all associated with loneliness.

Many interventions aim to reduce social isolation or loneliness in older people.[39–41] Common features of effective interventions were those developed within the context of a theoretic basis, those offering social activity or support within a group format, and those requiring active participation.[41] MacLeod[39] classified interventions into 1 of 4 categories: (1) telephone-based interventions; (2) community involvement; (3) online and digital solutions; and (4) resilience training. Each type of intervention has examples of success, but evidence often was not rigorous. Internet training interventions were effective only 25% of the time.[41]

The AARP has created significant capacity to advance this work.[45] Its comprehensive framework document identifies several community-based approaches with documented success. Examples include local departments of aging, Administration for Community Living, and US Administration on Aging. Palo Alto Medical Foundation and Commonwealth Fund created an innovative community-based collaboration.[46] Ultimately, the available data do not support a single best approach to this problem but many successful interventions are available as models for interested clinicians.

COMMUNITY HEALTH WORKERS AND PREVENTION

A community health worker (CHW) is a "frontline public health worker who is a trusted member of and/or has an unusually close understanding of the community served. ... serves as a liaison/link/intermediary between health/social services and the community ... also builds individual and community capacity by increasing health knowledge and self-sufficiency through a range of activities...."[47] CHWs may augment primary prevention or disease management services. Programs that target people with chronic diseases identify people at higher risk of other diseases. For example, programs aimed at improving hypertension control would be expected to reduce the burden of cardiovascular disease.

In the United States, health care organizations have collaborated with CHWs to create community-clinical linkages.[48] Examples of successful CHW programs elsewhere in the world include maternal and child health, infectious disease prevention, and cardiovascular disease prevention by managing hypertension.[49] Factors that facilitate success of CHWs include community embeddedness (with community members having a sense of ownership of the program), supportive supervision (often from health care organizations), continuous education, and adequate logistical support and supplies.[50]

Although the cost-effectiveness of CHW programs is inconsistent, some randomized trials of CHW interventions have shown impressive results. Provision of in-home asthma self-management support by CHWs to low-income adults with uncontrolled asthma improved asthma control and quality of life but not unscheduled health care use.[51] When compared with a control group with goal setting, a CHW intervention in patients who resided in a high-poverty zip code, were uninsured or publicly insured, and who had a diagnosis for 2 or more chronic diseases was associated with significant positive effects of patients' perceived quality of care, 30-day hospital readmissions, and overall hospital utilization.[52]

There are more than 50 published studies of CHWs working with people with T2D.[53,54] Patients with poorly controlled blood sugar are more likely to benefit from CHW support than patients with better glycemic control. The principal roles of CHWs are education, support, and advocacy. Training curricula for the role are available from the American Diabetes Association and the National Diabetes Education Program.

A collaboration of the El Paso, Texas Parks and Recreation Department, YWCA, and Centro San Vicente, a community health clinic, used 3 Promotoras de Salud to deliver services aimed at improving cardiovascular disease risk factors.[55] The intervention was associated with improvements in health behaviors and cardiovascular risk factors, with more favorable changes associated with great utilization of community resources.

SUMMARY

The health care landscape is changing as value-based payment models gain popularity with payers, policy makers, and health care organizations. These models share a goal of cost containment and most are predicated on improving the health of populations. Although modification of behavioral, social, and environmental factors has not historically been a core expectation of primary care, shifting from volume-based to value-based payment will drive increased accountability for disease prevention and thus growing interest in social and behavioral determinants of health. This opens opportunities for better partnerships with public health agencies, other community-based organizations, and the redefining of team-based primary care, as discussed in this article.

Health care organizations aiming to improve the health of populations via new payment models should pay attention to growing health disparities. Although many interventions target underserved populations who bear a disproportionate share of disease burden, there exists a risk of health care organizations increasing disparities if the higher potential revenue from commercial payers diverts attention away from low-income or other vulnerable populations. Thus, health care organizations should be very intentional with strategies to measure and mitigate health care disparities as part of their overall population-based approach to health promotion and disease prevention.

Finally, it is imperative to emphasize the role of prevention, public health, and policy in preventing disease. Rose's last sentence of *Preventive Medicine* reads, "the primary determinants of disease are mainly economic and social, and therefore its remedies must also be economic and social. Medicine and politics cannot and should not be kept apart."[2] The success of value-based payment models in improving population health will depend substantially on aligning local and national policies to improve social and environmental determinants of health.

ACKNOWLEDGMENTS

The authors gratefully acknowledge helpful input about this article from our colleagues at the University of Washington, Jeffrey R. Harris, MD, MPH, MBA, and Peggy A. Hannon, PhD, MPH.

REFERENCES

1. Schroeder SA. We can do better – improving the health of the American people. N Engl J Med 2007;357(12):1221–8.
2. Rose GA, Khaw K-T, Marmot MG. Rose's strategy of preventive medicine: the complete original text. Oxford (England): Oxford University Press; 2008.
3. Frieden TR. A framework for public health action: the health impact pyramid. Am J Public Health 2010;100(4):590–5.
4. Maciosek MV, Coffield AB, Edwards NM, et al. Priorities among effective clinical preventive services results of a systematic review and analysis. Am J Prev Med 2006;31(1):52–61.
5. Maciosek MV, Coffield AB, Flottemesch TJ, et al. Greater use of preventive services in U.S. health care could save lives at little or no cost. Health Aff 2010; 29(9):1656–60.
6. Farley TA, Dalal MA, Mostashari F, et al. Deaths preventable in the U.S. by improvements in use of clinical preventive services. Am J Prev Med 2010;38(6): 600–9.
7. Bodenheimer T, Ghorob A, Willard-Grace R, et al. The 10 building blocks of high-performing primary care. Ann Fam Med 2014;12(2):166–71.
8. Coronado GD, Petrik AF, Vollmer WM, et al. Effectiveness of a mailed colorectal cancer screening outreach program in community health clinics: the STOP CRC cluster randomized clinical trial. JAMA Intern Med 2018;178(9):1174–81.
9. Brenner AT, Rhode J, Yang JY, et al. Comparative effectiveness of mailed reminders with and without fecal immunochemical tests for Medicaid beneficiaries at a large county health department: a randomized controlled trial. Cancer 2018; 124(16):3346–54.
10. Ghorob A. Health coaching: teaching patients to fish. Fam Pract Manag 2013; 20(3):40–2.
11. Goldman ML, Ghorob A, Hessler D, et al. Are low-income peer health coaches able to master and utilize evidence-based health coaching? Ann Fam Med 2015;13(Suppl 1):S36–41.
12. Sherifali D, Viscardi V, Bai JW, et al. Evaluating the effect of a diabetes health coach in individuals with type 2 diabetes. Can J Diabetes 2016;40(1):84–94.
13. Crittenden D, Seibenhener S, Hamilton B. Health coaching and the management of hypertension. J Nurs Pract 2017;13(5):e237–9.
14. Willard-Grace R, Chen EH, Hessler D, et al. Health coaching by medical assistants to improve control of diabetes, hypertension, and hyperlipidemia in low-income patients: a randomized controlled trial. Ann Fam Med 2015;13(2):130–8.

15. Thom DH, Willard-Grace R, Tsao S, et al. Randomized controlled trial of health coaching for vulnerable patients with chronic obstructive pulmonary disease. Ann Am Thorac Soc 2018;15(10):1159–68.

16. Thom DH, Hessler D, Willard-Grace R, et al. Does health coaching change patients' trust in their primary care provider? Patient Educ Couns 2014;96(1):135–8.

17. Johnson C, Saba G, Wolf J, et al. What do health coaches do? Direct observation of health coach activities during medical and patient-health coach visits at 3 federally qualified health centers. Patient Educ Couns 2018;101(5):900–7.

18. Downing J, Bollyky J, Schneider J. Use of a connected glucose meter and certified diabetes educator coaching to decrease the likelihood of abnormal blood glucose excursions: The Livongo for Diabetes program. J Med Internet Res 2017;19(7):e234.

19. Bollyky J, Bravata D, Yang J, et al. Remote lifestyle coaching plus a connected glucose meter with certified diabetes educator support improves glucose and weight loss for people with type 2 diabetes. J Diabetes Res 2018;2018:3961730.

20. Chiguluri V, Barthold D, Gumpina R, et al. Virtual diabetes prevention program— Effects on Medicare Advantage health care costs and utilization. Diabetes 2018; 67(suppl 1). https://doi.org/10.2337/db18-45-lb.

21. DeJonghe LAL, Beckera J, Froboesea I, et al. Long-term effectiveness of health coaching in rehabilitation and prevention: a systematic review. Patient Educ Couns 2017;100(9):1643–53.

22. Porterfield DS, Hinnant LW, Kane H, et al. Linkages between clinical practices and community organizations for prevention: a literature review and environmental scan. Am J Public Health 2012;102:S375–82.

23. Centers for Disease Control and Prevention. Community-clinical linkages for the prevention and control of chronic diseases: a practitioner's guide. Atlanta (GA): Centers for Disease Control and Prevention, U.S. Department of Health and Human Services; 2016.

24. American Diabetes Association. The staggering cost of diabetes. Available at: http://www.diabetes.org/diabetes-basics/statistics/infographics/adv-staggering-cost-of-diabetes.html. Accessed December 21, 2018.

25. Knowler WC, Barrett-Connor E, Fowler SE, et al. Reduction in the incidence of type 2 diabetes with lifestyle intervention or metformin. N Engl J Med 2002; 346(6):393–403.

26. Knowler WC, Fowler SE, Hamman RF, et al. 10-year follow-up of diabetes incidence and weight loss in the Diabetes Prevention Program Outcomes Study. Lancet 2009;374(9702):1677–86.

27. Ackermann RT, Marrero DG. Adapting the diabetes prevention program lifestyle intervention for delivery in the community: the YMCA model. Diabetes Educ 2007; 33(1):69–78.

28. Ackermann RT, Liss DT, Finch EA, et al. A randomized comparative effectiveness trial for preventing type 2 diabetes. Am J Public Health 2015;105:2328–34.

29. Centers for Disease Control and Prevention. Diabetes Prevention Recognition Program – Registry of Recognized Organizations. Available at: https://nccd.cdc.gov/DDT_DPRP/Registry.aspx. Accessed October 15, 2018.

30. Alva ML, Hoerger TJ, Jeyaraman R, et al. Impact of the YMCA of the USA diabetes prevention program on Medicare spending and utilization. Health Aff 2017;36(3):417–24.

31. Physical activity Guidelines for Americans, 2nd edition. Available at: https://health.gov/paguidelines/second-edition/. Accessed November 21, 2018.

32. American College of Sports Medicine. Exercise is Medicine. Available at: https://www.exerciseismedicine.org/support_page.php/about-eim5/. Accessed November 21, 2018.

33. National physical activity plan. 2016. Available at: http://www.physicalactivityplan.org/theplan/about.html. Accessed November 23, 2018.

34. CDC Physical Activity Guidelines. Implementation Resources Guide. Available at: https://www.cdc.gov/physicalactivity/community-strategies/beactive/implementation-resource-guide.html. Accessed November 23, 2018.

35. Wolfenden L, Goldman S, Stacey FG, et al. Strategies to improve the implementation of workplace-based policies or practices targeting tobacco, alcohol, diet, physical activity and obesity. Cochrane Database Syst Rev 2018;(11):CD012439.

36. Greenwood-Hickman MA, Rosenberg DE, Phelan EA, et al. Participation in older adult physical activity programs and risk for falls requiring medical care, Washington State, 2005–2011. Prev Chronic Dis 2015;12:140574.

37. Wallace JI, Buchner DM, Grothaus L, et al. Implementation and effectiveness of a community-based health promotion program for older adults. J Gerontol A Biol Sci Med Sci 1998;53(4):M301–6.

38. Sound Generations. Welcome to Project Enhance. Available at: http://www.projectenhance.org/. Accessed November 23, 2018.

39. MacLeod S. Examining approaches to address loneliness and social isolation among older adults. Journal of Aging and Geriatric Medicine 2018;2:1.

40. Masi CM, Chen HY, Hawkley LC, et al. A meta-analysis of interventions to reduce loneliness. Pers Soc Psychol Rev 2011;15(3):219–66.

41. Dickens AP, Richards SH, Greaves CJ, et al. Interventions targeting social isolation in older people: a systematic review. BMC Public Health 2011;11:647.

42. Theeke LA. Predictors of loneliness in U.S. adults over age sixty-five. Arch Psychiatr Nurs 2009;23(5):387–96.

43. Perissinotto CM, Stijacic Cenzer I, Covinsky KE. Loneliness in older persons: a predictor of functional decline and death. Arch Intern Med 2012;172(14): 1078–83.

44. Musich S, Wang SS, Hawkins K, et al. The impact of loneliness on quality of life and patient satisfaction among older, sicker adults. Gerontol Geriatr Med 2015;1–9. https://doi.org/10.1177/2333721415582119.

45. AARP Foundation. Framework for isolation in adults over 50. Washington, DC: 2012.

46. Hayes SL, McCarthy D, Klein S. Linkages: building support systems for seniors living independently in the community. New York: Commonwealth Fund; 2015.

47. American Public Health Association. Community health workers. 2016. Available at: https://www.apha.org/apha-communities/member-sections/community-health-workers. Accessed November 19, 2018.

48. Lohr AM, Ingram M, Nuñez AV, et al. Community–clinical linkages with community health workers in the United States: a scoping review. Health Promot Pract 2018; 19(3):349–60.

49. Vaughan K, Kok MC, Witter S, et al. Costs and cost-effectiveness of community health workers: evidence from a literature review. Hum Resour Health 2015;13: 71–87.

50. Scott K, Beckham SW, Gross M, et al. What do we know about community-based health worker programs? A systematic review of existing reviews on community health workers. Hum Resour Health 2018;16:39–56.

51. Krieger J, Song L, Philby M. Community health worker home visits for adults with uncontrolled asthma. The HomeBASE Trial randomized clinical trial. JAMA Intern Med 2015;175(1):109–17.
52. Kangovi S, Mitra N, Norton L, et al. Effect of community health worker support on clinical outcomes of low-income patients across primary care facilities. A randomized clinical trial. JAMA Intern Med 2018;178(12):1635–43.
53. Egbujie BA, Delobelle PA, Levitt N, et al. Role of community health workers in type 2 diabetes mellitus self-management: a scoping review. PLoS One 2018;13(6): e0198424.
54. Palmas W, March D, Darakjy S, et al. Community health worker interventions to improve glycemic control in people with diabetes: A systematic review and meta-analysis. J Gen Intern Med 2015;30(7):1004–12.
55. De Heer HD, Balcazar HG, Wise S, et al. Improved cardiovascular risk among Hispanic border participants of the Mi Corazón Mi Comunidad Promotores de Salud Model: the HEART II cohort intervention study 2009–2013. Front Public Health 2015;3:149–56.

Quality Improvement Principles and Practice

Shana Ratner, MD[a],*, Michael Pignone, MD, MPH, MACP[b]

KEYWORDS

- Quality improvement • Care transformation • Rapid cycle improvement
- Primary care • Patient engagement

KEY POINTS

- Implementing quality improvement processes can improve care and increase provider satisfaction.
- Starting small is important: begin with easier projects and use small tests of change to work out processes, and then focus on sustainment and spread.
- Effective improvement requires input from all members of the care team, and ideally from patients as well.
- Making a current process map is an important early step to improvement, and can suggest appropriate targets for change.
- Collecting data is essential to improvement, and often can be done on a small scale, especially early in an improvement process.

INTRODUCTION: HOW CAN QUALITY IMPROVEMENT SKILLS BE HELPFUL IN PRIMARY CARE PRACTICE? (IE, WHY SHOULD YOU READ THIS?)

A quality improvement strategy has become increasingly recognized as an essential ingredient for the success of health care organizations. Those who work in health care settings may benefit from developing skills and experience in quality improvement in several ways: foremost, quality improvement skills enable provision of a higher quality of care and can increase value (quality of care divided by cost). In addition, the authors have found that engaging in quality improvement can improve job satisfaction and reduce frustration and symptoms of burnout by helping providers become more engaged in care processes. Done well, quality improvement is also more nimble than

Disclosure: The authors have nothing to disclose.
[a] Department of Medicine, Division of General Internal Medicine and Clinical Epidemiology, University of North Carolina Chapel Hill, 5034 Old Clinic Building, CB 7110, Chapel Hill, NC 27599, USA; [b] Department of Internal Medicine, Dell Medical School, University of Texas, DMS Health Discovery Building, Room 7.704, 1701 Trinity Street, Stop Z0900, Austin, TX 78712-1876, USA
* Corresponding author.
E-mail address: shana_ratner@med.unc.edu

Prim Care Clin Office Pract 46 (2019) 505–514
https://doi.org/10.1016/j.pop.2019.07.008
0095-4543/19/© 2019 Elsevier Inc. All rights reserved.

primarycare.theclinics.com

other methods, such as traditional clinical or health services research, for understanding systematically how to deliver better care. This article outlines some key principles that enable successful quality improvement, based on our experiences in large, academic health systems and their community affiliates.

GETTING STARTED: HOW TO IDENTIFY GOOD PROJECTS

When starting quality improvement work, teams should consider brainstorming and discussing their biggest frustrations in daily practice, particularly ones that they perceive affect patients' quality of care. Starting with problems that are salient and common can help build engagement. Building engagement increases buy-in for the hard work of change in the future. The hope is that by deeply engaging in the work of improving pain points in their work, job satisfaction may increase, thus building momentum and increasing engagement. The authors have seen in our experiences that increasing provider engagement and self-efficacy can reduce burnout, improve engagement, and perhaps decrease turnover. Stories about lapses in patient care, quality, and safety are the most compelling burning platform to motivate our work.

In a practice's improvement journey, it can be helpful to start with problems that lend themselves well to easy wins, particularly in cases in which the interventions to overcome care deficits are straightforward and not complex. This strategy helps the team build change management capabilities as well as self-efficacy and excitement. For instance, an improvement team in primary care may want to start with improving pneumococcal vaccination rates, an easy care gap to address, as opposed to blood pressure control, which is a much more complex process of identification and treatment. As teams have initial successes, begin to gain confidence, and see their work improving care, they will be able to successfully take on more complex issues.

In picking a project, clinical units that are part of larger organizations need to balance internal needs versus larger institutional goals and objectives. Ideally, there is an overlap between these two. If the overlap is not obvious, teams may also consider modifying their local initiatives to match system-wide efforts. For example, locally identified efforts to improve access to appointments for acutely ill patients can be linked with system goals to reduce readmissions through timely postdischarge follow-up visits.

There is a tremendous amount of waste and inefficiency in medicine, and many recent efforts have been directed at waste reduction.[1] However, teams often find that focusing solely on waste or cost reduction is a less effective motivator for the teams, especially at first. The authors have found most success by starting with efforts to improve some care process that increase the underuse of an effective service, one that can be closely linked with patient health outcomes. In our experience, teams find and reduce waste and inefficiency while working to improve outcomes for patients, even without it being the primary focus.

FORMING A TEAM

Quality improvement is a "team sport." Most important care processes in primary care (and most other settings) involve multiple care team members, as well as the patient and the patient's family. As such, the only way clinicians can expect to improve outcomes is to engage multiple members of the clinical team in the improvement effort. The definition of the care team needs to be expanded to include members who have traditionally not been thought of as having direct care responsibilities, including those who receive and direct phone calls within a practice, custodial staff, and community health workers.[2]

In addition to engaging diverse members of the care team, it is helpful to include a patient/family advisor in the team as well.[3] Including a patient or family member from the beginning helps to ensure that patient perspectives are taken into account and keep the team accountable to why they are doing this work. Large institutions may already have a patient and family advisory board made up of individuals who have been selected and prepared for this work. In other cases, practices may wish to form their own advisory panels.

For example, in our colorectal cancer screening work the authors included administrative assistants who make phone calls, nurses who give out stool tests and educate patients, physicians, advanced practice providers, patients, representatives from gastroenterology, and care managers.

Practice managers and leaders should act as sponsors and be informed about the progress of improvement efforts so they can remove barriers and facilitate time for the team to meet. However, they do not necessarily need to be represented on every improvement team, particularly as the practice gains more experience and wishes to conduct multiple efforts simultaneously.

BUILDING MOMENTUM FOR IMPROVEMENT

Once the practice has selected an area on which to work and formed an improvement team, the authors have found patient stories to be an effective means of building interest and engagement across the practice. A compelling patient story about a quality or safety gap helps bring out the true intrinsic motivation of the team and helps move them to action. Ideally, such stories also help build a "burning platform" for improvement. A burning platform implies that the current state cannot be continued, and that change is required. Creating a sense of the need for change can help overcome inertia and the natural tendency to replicate the status quo. In building momentum for change, having quantitative data is important, but, in our experience, sharing data alone is less effective than also including a compelling story: developing and communicating compelling stories is a skill that requires practice.

DEFINING THE PROBLEM AND SETTING GOALS

One barrier that seems to impede progress in improvement work is overthinking how to define the problem. The authors have observed teams spending months debating which guideline to follow or worrying about exactly how to define a metric or goal for improvement. Prolonged planning can derail improvement teams and squander momentum, especially for less experienced teams. We advise teams to try to choose a nationally agreed-on quality metric, recognizing that it may not be perfect but is often good enough. In terms of setting specific goals, we have found it important to emphasize directional and short-term change goals, rather than focusing on what would be considered ideal. Returning to the colon cancer screening example, once we identified our performance in the nationally agreed-on measure of current screening (by any recommended method) to be in the 60% range, we set a short-term (12 month) goal of increasing it to 65%, rather than setting the initial goal at 80%, a level many national entities had espoused as an (eventual) goal.[4,5]

CREATING A PROJECT PLAN

Once sufficient energy for change has been developed and a reasonable problem and goal defined, teams can progress to creating a project plan or charter. The charter (**Fig. 1**) is a brief (1–3 page) document that captures the nature of the problem, its

PROBLEM STATEMENT

The colorectal cancer (CRC) screening rate for patients seen in the Internal Medicine Clinic (IMC) during 2011–2012 was 63%. The current process used in IMC designed to lead patients to receiving a CRC screening has resulted in 2728 defects (or missed opportunities) out of 7337 opportunities in 2011–2012. The CRC Screening process used in IMC needs to be improved in order to reduce the number of missed opportunities.

IMPORTANCE STATEMENT

CRC is the second leading cause of cancer-related death in the United States. CRC screening can detect premalignant polyps and early stage cancers. Removal of premalignant polyps can decrease incidence of CRC. Detecting and treating early stage cancers may improve associated morbidity and mortality, and lower costs.

Beyond the importance to patient care, CRC screening rates are a measure in the Physician Quality Reporting System Group Practice Reporting Option for which performance measures will be publicly available beginning in 2013 and will likely impact reimbursement beginning in 2015. The performance measure for the group practice (45.3% for 2011) will be applied to all UNCFP UNC Faculty Physicians, formerly P&A)physicians. This rate is lower than those reported by other group practices (mean = 57%, 90th percentile = 74%).

It is a FY13 UNC Health Care organizational goal to increase CRC screening rates by 10%. Since primary care physicians are most likely to order CRC screening, increasing the screening rate for IMC patients is expected to increase the overall UNC P&A rate.

SCOPE

In Scope: CRC screening processes at the IMC	Out of Scope: CRC screening processes at other clinics
Start (first step): Office visit scheduled	End (last step): Colonoscopy or other screening method documented

Fig. 1. Project charter. FY13, fiscal year 2013; P&A, physicians and associates; UNC, University of North Carolina; UNCFP, University of North Carolina Faculty Physician.

importance, and the measures to be used. Ideally, a multidisciplinary team creates this chartering document. The process of creating it is as important as the content.

CARRYING OUT IMPROVEMENT

Improving outcomes in health care is most often accomplished by clarifying, streamlining, simplifying, and improving care processes. The authors hypothesize that part of the growing burnout epidemic in health care arises from health care providers knowing what needs to be done to help their patients, but facing many barriers to how to get the key work done. Patient factors, system factors, time pressures, and competing demands often preclude achieving the best outcomes. Identifying and breaking down these barriers leads to improved clinical outcomes as well as increased provider and patient satisfaction. Some of the helpful tools to aid in process improvement are summarized here.

UNDERSTANDING THE CURRENT STATE: PROCESS MAPPING

In developing plans for how to perform improvement, the first key step is to better understand the current state. One effective means is for the team to create a process map (**Fig. 2**). In process mapping, the team works together to identify all of the steps that go into a process, including all of the decision points. In general, the more steps and decision points noted in a process, the more likely that process is to fail. The act of creating a process map can be highly revealing; team members may identify complexity in the process of which they were not even aware, or misconceptions about what is required to get the task done. It is often illuminating to see how many workarounds and redundancies there can be in seemingly straightforward care processes. The most important aspect of process mapping is having the frontline staff create the process map showing the reality of the process. This real process map is often different from what leadership imagines it to be.

Process mapping does not require any sophisticated technology. The map can simply be drawn out on paper. The authors often place each step on a sticky note on a

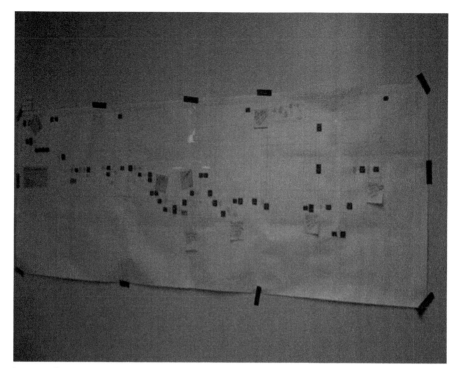

Fig. 2. Colonoscopy process map.

large wall or piece of paper, and then move the individual sticky notes around as we learn more and clarify the process. The team can investigate and go deeper if there are uncertainties about the details of the process. Returning to our colon cancer screening example, the authors developed separate process maps for stool testing and colonoscopy. At the time, we realized that there were 71 steps or decisions to complete stool testing and 75 steps to complete colonoscopy. It was no wonder we were not getting the consistent screening results we desired.

To most effectively identify the care processes, it is necessary to "go to the Gemba." In the terminology of Lean methodology, the Gemba is the place of truth where the work is done. Going to the Gemba involves physically walking the care environment and talking to frontline staff about how the key processes work. In our example, we visited the laboratory where stool cards are processed for colon cancer screening, walked around the clinic and talked to the nurses, and saw where they obtain stool tests. It might also mean going to the gastrointestinal clinic and talking to its referral coordinators about the process that occurs when they receive an order for a colonoscopy. It should also include talking with patients about how they experience all aspects of the testing process, including the return of results.

DRIVER DIAGRAM

Another tool teams can use is a driver diagram (**Fig. 3**). This tool helps break down the problem into different categories and pieces, facilitating identification of key themes for improvement.[6] The act of working together and creating this diagram can spark conversation and communication between team members, which can illuminate

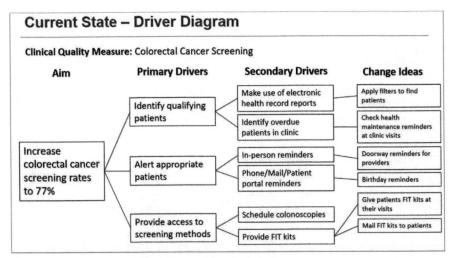

Fig. 3. Driver diagram. FIT, fecal immunochemical testing.

root causes or barriers to improvement. This process can make the problem seem more "bite size" and suggests potential discrete changes that can be addressed for improvement. When teams create driver diagrams, they often realize there will not be 1 overarching "magic bullet" to fix the issue, but instead multiple different smaller opportunities for change and improvement.

CONDUCTING SMALL TESTS OF CHANGE

The most important step a quality improvement team can take is to start small, purposeful tests of elements of a new process. These small tests of change are commonly called PDSA(plan/do/study/act) or PDCA cycles (plan/do/ check/act).

A common misconception about PDSAs is that a team would do months of planning, then roll out a well-thought-out intervention to the whole clinic population for a few months, then measure the outcomes and decide what to do next.

We have found it is much more powerful to do small iterations of the process. We recommend starting small with 1 patient, 1 provider, and 1 staff member, and a single day. Try out the new process. Get feedback from everyone (including the patient). Look for the problems, inefficiencies, and frustrations, and then change something to improve it. Then try it again that afternoon or the next day in the new way. Do this over and over again with increasingly better versions of the intervention. Make sure all stakeholders are involved and receiving feedback. Then start to scale up from 1 clinician and 1 nurse to 3 clinicians and 3 nurses, then 10, and so forth.

By doing the initial PDSAs with a small, engaged group, the team is able to learn and improve faster. When the more perfected intervention starts to roll out to a larger group, many of the kinks will have been worked out.

In the initial PDSAs, the team does not need reports or technological analytics. All of the initial small process measures are often things the team can count with simple tick marks and subjective feedback. How many times did it get done, how many missed opportunities were there, what was the feedback? What were the pain points?

An example from our work of how small a PDSA can be is when our clinic was switching from guaiac-based fecal occult blood testing (gFOBT) to fecal immuno-chemical testing (FIT) as our stool-based method of colon cancer screening. A student working on the improvement team sat down with a nurse to try to create 1 new FIT kit to give to patients. This process involved getting the proper order, patient label, testing kit, and return envelope, and then placing the return address to the laboratory on the envelope. When the student and nurse sat down to make 1 kit as part of a PDSA cycle, they attempted to use the same return address stamp previously used for gFOBT kits. This step seems negligible. However, when they stamped the new FIT kit envelope, it turned out the envelope was shiny instead of matte, and the return address stamp wiped right off. This pitfall is something that would never have been discovered around a conference table, even with all of the right stakeholders in the room. It was only by testing our new process that we uncovered this problem and then came up with a (simple) strategy to solve it. Had the team started with a big roll-out on day 1 and made and sent 200 kits to patients, imagine the frustration patients and staff would have felt about the new process.

The authors find it can be helpful to track PDSAs and see how many iterations or tests we can do. We use low-tech solutions such as paper forms that we can modify from patient to patient or day to day. We have learned not to laminate anything until tested with many stakeholders through many iterations.

CREATING AND SUSTAINING A CULTURE OF IMPROVEMENT

Once a practice gains facility with identifying problems, selecting and prioritizing issues, and conducting PDSA cycles to test potential improvements, it begins to build a track record of improvement and develop a cadre of providers with expertise in this area. Once such skills are established, the next challenge is to sustain them through building a culture of improvement.

CREATING VISUAL MANAGEMENT SYSTEMS

One key feature of organizations with advanced improvement cultures is transparency of data. Such practices post their aggregate quality data and lessons learned where all can see, including patients. Visual management boards (**Fig. 4**) display process and outcome data and make clear that the team is transparent and open about improvement. Everyone can study them and know how the unit is doing, what the goal is, and whether they are moving in the right direction.

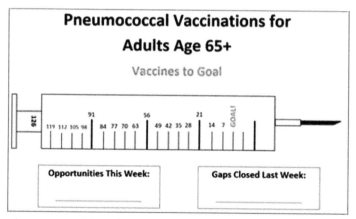

Fig. 4. Visual management board

This visual management board is used in clinics to track the number of pneumonia vaccines to be given to reach an agreed-on goal. This board was posted in a public area. The team could visualize their progress and track opportunities in real time.

SHARING AND FEEDING BACK DATA

One question in sharing performance data is whether performance should be measured and shared at the individual provider or team level. Practices with advanced improvement cultures generally find that sharing data at the level of the functional team can help spur additional progress. Such data should not be used to shame or punish providers who are underperforming. Instead, teams can practice so-called bright spotting,[7] identifying those with high performance, and humbly asking what are they doing well that is leading to these exceptional results. The intent should be to identify best practices that can be spread to others.[8,9]

When the authors were beginning our work on improving colorectal cancer screenings, we obtained and reviewed our providers' individual data. We found 1 physician whose performance far exceeded others'. We informally asked her how she approached the problem. She shared with us how she talked to patients about screening (scripting), how she approached shared decision making with patients, and how she worked to obtain outside records when tests were done elsewhere. We shared these insights with others and worked to build systems to hardwire these approaches into the care that was being provided.

One common pitfall of overemphasizing provider-level data is focusing on individual physician results when the best pathway to improvement is not at the level of the physician. A common example is that of immunizations: in high-functioning clinic teams, there are standing orders so that medical assistants or nurses can give vaccinations based on protocols without requiring a new individual order from a physician or advanced practice provider for each care episode. However, provider-level quality data rarely identify the care team doing the work but instead give the provider credit or blame.

The authors have found it is best initially to share performance data in a face-to-face meeting. This way, leaders can explain how they will use the data and how improvement will be approached, focusing on bright spotting and opportunities to learn. When data are shared, there is often a tendency to focus on limitations in the data. It is important for leaders to ensure the data that is shared is accurate, while also acknowledging that data are not perfect, and lack of perfect data should not paralyze change. Individuals should be encouraged to report when they see discrepancies in the data, so steps can be taken to make the reports better. Providing time for discussion can help improve buy-in into this process. On a monthly basis, we email data out to the whole practice (providers, nurses, medical assistants, front desk staff). We highlight improvements and opportunities and take time to celebrate top-performing teams. We also post the data on a board in our clinic.

Many leaders believe that the process of measuring and feeding back performance data (audit and feedback) is enough to produce improvement. The authors have found that audit and feedback alone are not particularly effective for sustaining improvement; however, they can serve as one impetus to examining the care process and identifying key structural barriers (and key bright spots of innovation) that can be used to drive and spread improvement through rapid cycle improvement processes.

CELEBRATION

It is important that practices and clinical units take the time to celebrate successes and discuss opportunities for further growth. The authors have found many practical ways to do this. At our quarterly practice all-hands meeting, we celebrate individuals and teams with high quality and patient satisfaction scores, emphasizing patient stories gleaned from our satisfaction surveys. In addition, we recognize those who have participated in quality improvement teams. We recognize on boards in the clinics the top performers for the week or month, which drives friendly competition and tends to increase motivation. We have also sought ways to reward group efforts. For instance, setting a team goal and providing a lunch or party when the team reaches their goal is an appreciated reward.

We seek not only to celebrate successes but also to celebrate instances in which we observe that the attempted improvement fails. As leaders, we embrace the model of "fail faster," encouraging our teams to try their own PDSAs to see what processes work in their settings, and to perceive cases in which the innovation failed as a "victory of learning."

SHARED LEARNING/COLLABORATIVES

In addition to clinicians sharing within their own practices, joining a group of practices in a learning collaborative (whether local, regional, or national) can accelerate improvement and change. Learning collaboratives offer the opportunity to bring together groups of likeminded individuals to share experiences (both positive and negative) and build community. Practices can start by forming a collaborative with 1 other practice, then build up to larger, more diverse collaborations.

SUSTAINMENT

Although teams often do great work improving quality and care, these efforts are at risk of not being sustained once start-up energy and project-specific resources are exhausted. There are several keys to improving the likelihood of sustainability.

Foremost, a major key to sustainment is considering it from the start of the project. By including frontline staff in the decision making and as members of the team, changes will be self-imposed and designed to work within existing workflows, as opposed to being perceived as an external mandate. Once PDSAs have helped determine a workable and successful method of doing the new process, teams can build out a standard work document and define a process owner. The process owner is responsible for ensuring that new members of the care team are trained in this process, that it is reviewed and updated periodically, and that someone is looking at data to ensure that the process is continuing to produce desired results.

SUMMARY

This article outlines several key lessons learned from our work in building a robust quality improvement program within primary care practices. Key points include starting small, ideally with a care process that is not too complex; engaging a diverse team; striving to understand the current state through process mapping; developing a project charter and driver diagram; using multiple small tests of change to improve the process; the importance of celebrating success and sharing data; and recognizing the importance of sustainability early in the improvement process. Although these principles have been developed through a wide range of improvement work, there is still much to learn about how best to encourage a culture of improvement, and the authors encourage those engaged in improvement work to share their successes and learning broadly.

ACKNOWLEDGMENTS

Christina McMillan; Christine Gladman, MD, MPH; Brooke McGuirt, MBA; Jonathan Thornhill, MHA, MS; Patrick Notini, MD; Thomas Lunsford, MD for their involvement and engagement with this work.

REFERENCES

1. Available at: www.choosingwisely.org. Accessed September 10, 2019.
2. Available at: http://www.ihi.org/resources/Pages/HowtoImprove/ScienceofImprovementFormingtheTeam.aspx. Accessed September 10, 2019.
3. Guide to patient and family engagement in hospital quality and safety. Content last reviewed December. Rockville (MD): Agency for Healthcare Research and Quality; 2017. Available at: http://www.ahrq.gov/professionals/systems/hospital/engagingfamilies/guide.html.
4. National colorectal cancer roundtable. Available at: http://nccrt.org/. Accessed September 10, 2019.
5. Meester RGS, Doubeni CA, Zauber AG, et al. Public health impact of achieving 80% colorectal cancer screening rates in the United States by 2018. Cancer 2015;121:2281–5.
6. Bennett B, Provost L. What's your theory? Qual Prog 2015;2:37–43.
7. Heath C, Heath D. Switch: how to change things when change is hard. New York: Broadway Books; 2010. Print.
8. Hysong S, Best R, Pugh J. Audit and feedback and clinical practice guideline adherence: making feedback actionable. Implement Sci 2006;1:9. Available at: www.implementationscience.com/content/1/1/9.
9. Jamtvedt G, Young JM, Kristoffersen DT, et al. Audit and feedback: effects on professional practice and health care outcomes. Cochrane Database Syst Rev 2006;(2). CD000259. Available at: https://www.cochranelibrary.com/cdsr/doi/10.1002/14651858.CD000259.pub3/full.

Lean Thinking for Primary Care

John B. Anderson, MD, MPH[a],*, Heather Marstiller, MBOE[b], Kevin Shah, MD, MBA[c]

KEYWORDS

- Lean thinking • Standard work • A3 thinking • Daily management system
- Visual management • Gemba visit • Leadership • PDSA

KEY POINTS

- Lean thinking involves focusing on continuous process improvement. Improvement is achieved through rigorous management of operational processes while avoiding management by results.
- Respect for people is critical to the success of any Lean endeavor. Those at the frontline, who actually perform the work, are best suited to solve the daily problems that are barriers to success.
- Lean will allow managers to move away from constant "fire-fighting" to deal with problems and move to a system of Standard Work that anticipates issues and deals with challenges proactively. Standard work allows leaders to have a deep understanding of their business and move problem solving down their leadership chain to those best suited to solve problems at the frontline.
- "A3" thinking involves an understanding of the current state with a clear definition of the problem one is trying to solve. It defines the ideal target state and the countermeasures to solve problems to root cause, overcome barriers, and continuously improve in alignment with the organization's "True North" goals.
- Creating a Lean Management System is critical to ensuring the success of any Lean transformation. Teaching leaders to behave differently ensures that this effort becomes the approach by which the organization is managed, rather than just another new initiative. Instead of problem solvers, leaders become coaches who help continuously develop improvement capabilities in managers and front-line staff.

WHAT IS LEAN?
Case Study

Betty Jo felt an increasing sense of dread as her 30-minute commute to work was ending. Early this morning she had received call-outs from 2 of her Medical Assistants,

Disclosure: The authors have nothing to disclose.
[a] Department of Family Medicine and Community Health, Duke Primary Care, Duke University Health System, 411 West Chapel Hill Street, Durham, NC 27701, USA; [b] Duke Primary Care, Duke University Health System, 411 West Chapel Hill Street, Durham, NC 27701, USA; [c] Department of Medicine, Duke Primary Care, Duke University Health System, 411 West Chapel Hill Street, Durham, NC 27701, USA
* Corresponding author.
E-mail address: john.anderson@duke.edu

Prim Care Clin Office Pract 46 (2019) 515–527
https://doi.org/10.1016/j.pop.2019.07.009
0095-4543/19/© 2019 Elsevier Inc. All rights reserved.

and she knew the office schedule was completely booked. Her providers routinely complained about the staffing shortages and their inability to stay on time. She had taken on the role of Practice Manager for Hillandale Family Medicine with the charge from her Chief Operating Officer of "turning this place around," but that was 3 months ago, and she was getting discouraged. Their quality metrics were below the network standards; their patient experience scores were not at target, and the providers were constantly voicing concerns about "burnout" and "work-life balance." Her days are spent constantly putting out fires and fixing everyone else's problems, while leaving no time for her other administrative tasks and the turnaround effort.

Lean operations in health care are based largely on the much-admired Toyota Production System and its application in manufacturing.[1] This approach migrated from Toyota to health care via several large health systems, including Virginia Mason in Seattle, Washington and ThedaCare in Appleton, Wisconsin. In Duke Primary Care, the authors have been using this approach to manage their daily operations and lead their continuous improvement efforts. These efforts help drive their success in improving population health metrics. In this article, the authors focus primarily on the Lean Management System and how it is critical to the support of their daily operations.

Lean is often thought of as a set of tools that one can use as part of project-based improvement work. Although these tools can be useful and are necessary to support a systems-based approach to operations, they are not sufficient for creating continuous improvement. It is important to understand a set of principles that underpins the culture required to build an organization that focuses on continuous improvement as a way of creating the greatest value for patients and staff. These principles (**Box 1**) are based on the work of the Shingo Institute currently housed at the University of Utah.[2]

Respect all individuals

It is critical that all people in the organization are treated with respect, including patients, staff, administration, and suppliers. Those closest to the work have the greatest understanding of how care is delivered and what the greatest barriers are. It is respectful to involve frontline providers, nurses, and medical assistants in solving problems and offering ideas for improvement. It is disrespectful to make patients wait and not involve them in their care. Respect for clinicians means they have appropriate staff and the necessary tools to deliver patient-centered care. Respect entails ensuring everyone understands the "why" just as much as they understand the "how."

Lead with humility

Leaders focus their attention on listening and learning rather than being directive and solving problems on their own. Their respect for individuals enables them to involve

---

Box 1
Lean principles

Respect all individuals

Lead with humility

Seek perfection

Embrace scientific thinking

Focus on process

Data from Utah State University. The Shingo model. Available at: https://www.shingo.org/model.

others in organizational improvement and humbly assume the role of facilitator and coach.

Seek perfection
The authors do not expect to achieve perfection, but it is in the pursuit of perfection that they are able to create a culture of continuous improvement. Seeking perfection means problems are solved at their root cause and that they are constantly looking for ways to simplify work, remove waste, and create efficiencies.

Embrace scientific thinking
Scientific thinking is the basis of the PDSA (Plan Do Study Act) approach to rapid, small tests of change that are linked to solve problems and create improvement. This approach allows individuals to learn from both failures and successes and ensures that only changes are made that result in measurable improvement.

Focus on process
All outcomes are created through a process. Ideal results occur through a systematic approach to continuous improvement of processes rather than forcing individuals to work harder and faster. When unable to meet the patients' needs or achieve expected targets, failure is often the result of poorly engineered processes rather than poorly performing individuals. The foundation of the ability to focus on process is called "standard work."

Putting these principles together creates the foundation on which to build the Lean Management "house" (**Fig. 1**).[3] The goal of leadership then becomes that of aligning these components in a systematic way to create engagement and enable the organization to achieve results that deliver the greatest value to patients and their families.

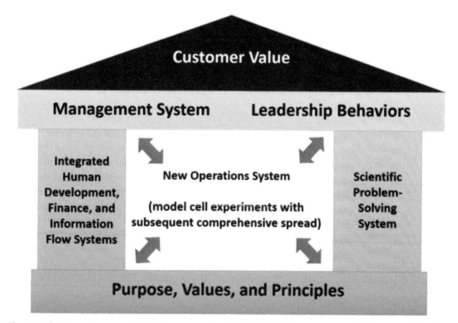

Fig. 1. The Lean management house. (*From* Catalysis. Systems approach for transforming healthcare organizations: improving the quality, cost, and value of patient care. Available at: https://createvalue.org/wp-content/uploads/Systems-Approach-for-Transforming-Healthcare-Organizations.pdf. Accessed Dec 28, 2018; with permission.)

Along the way, staff and providers feel valued for their work; there are opportunities for personal development, and the concept of "value-based care" has greater meaning.

Daily Management System

The creation of a daily management system is central to the creation of a culture that supports continuous improvement. It fosters a safe environment for staff to identify problems without fear of retribution, and it creates a forum to engage everyone in solving those problems. It creates a system that equates normal daily management with process improvement work, as opposed to viewing improvement as project based and separate from everyday management. As Mike Rother[4–6] reminds us in his book, *Toyota Kata*, our traditional approach is to focus on "outcome targets and consequences." In contrast, "Toyota puts considerable emphasis on how people tackle the details of a process, which is what generates the outcomes." Of course, outcomes are important, but with appropriate attention directed at improvement work, the outcomes will follow. A daily management system can be broken down into 6 components, as displayed in **Box 2**.

Teamlet daily huddles can occur wherever there are at least 2 individuals from a team. They are intended to be quick check-in activities that prepare participants for the day, follow up ongoing improvement work, and bring forward any new problems that are creating barriers to improvement. Providers should huddle with their medical assistant to review the day's schedule and take a proactive approach to the patients being seen that day. As examples, are there outside test results to track down, appropriate health maintenance interventions to schedule, immunizations to order, or medications that will need refilling?

The entire clinic team (providers, and clerical and clinical staff) huddles daily in front of the clinic Improvement Board (**Fig. 2**) to discuss what is needed to best prepare for the day and to support continued improvement. The huddle is also a time to celebrate success, raise safety concerns, use leading data to understand process performance, discuss improvement ideas, and review ongoing "work in progress." Team huddles are a great way to facilitate engagement of the entire staff and involve them in identifying problems. The authors have also used the huddle as a time to assess the "mood" of the office. Are people drowning in work, are they thriving, or are they stable? It is hard to engage in improvement work if everyone is feeling overwhelmed and just keeping their heads above water. This moment to assess the team mood is a daily practice of the Lean principle of respect. Daily huddles provide the team with the opportunity to submit new ideas for improvement and review ideas that have been suggested. The authors use a Pick chart to help prioritize ideas into quadrants that determine level of impact and degree of difficulty to implement. There is also an opportunity to decide which suggestions

---

Box 2
Six components of a daily management system

- Daily huddles
- Use of visual management
- Process observation
- Vitals Reports
- Standard work
- PDSA thinking

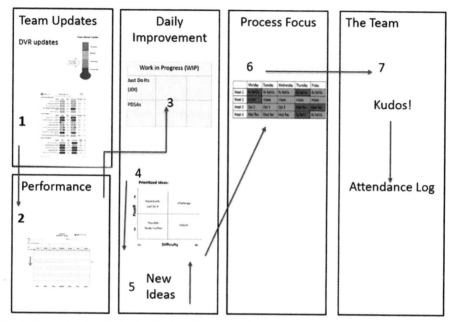

Fig. 2. Example of a Clinic Huddle Board. The numbers reflect a suggested order of review during the huddle. DVR, daily vitals reports.

fall into the "just-do-it" category. It is important to follow a standardized format to huddle that keeps everyone on task. Huddles should take no more than 10 to 15 minutes with everyone standing around the board and should not sidetrack the group by devolving into working on solutions. Finally, the huddle is also the opportunity to escalate problems further up the leadership chain that cannot be solved at the local level.

The use of visual management is an important component of any daily management system. The information informs the team and leaders of what is expected to happen versus what is actually happening, thereby allowing for real-time problem solving and adjustments. The use of visual tools that are displayed on Improvement Boards is meant to reflect ongoing improvement work and should paint a clear picture of what problems are being addressed through ongoing PDSA cycles. This system is not an opportunity to create "art on the wall" by posting fancy dashboards and charts of monthly performance results, but instead should be aligned with the hard work of solving problems and improving performance. Visual management creates a sense of transparency so anyone can see, at a rapid glance, the current state of affairs for that particular clinic or unit. It also creates a sense of accountability by making the work visible and indicating "by whom, by when" as part of the process.

Process observation is a useful tool that allows managers to check adherence to standard work and evaluate the need for improvement to the standard. Creating standard work hardwires a process so that it can be replicated and taught to others. It should reflect the most efficient way currently known to accomplish a task, which is necessary in order to improve. A process cannot be improved if it consists of multiple, chaotic workflows and is dependent on the individual rather than the standard. If there is deviation from standard work, staff is coached about their compliance or new opportunities for improvement are identified. It is also useful to make process

Table 1	
Vitals Report questions	
Metrics	Weekly Measures
Safety	• What safety concerns have we had this week? • What measures have we taken: Root Cause Analysis work? • Tell me about any updates on outstanding safety reports? • What building/facility/equipment issues have we had this week? • What barriers can I assist with to expedite resolution?
Quality	• What are the new PDSAs in the practice • What did you anticipate and prevent this week? • What did you go and see last week? What did you learn?
Service	• What areas are we not able to meet patient expectations? • What patient compliments have we had this week? • What are the Transforming Primary Care Collaborative standard work challenges for this week? • What solutions do you recommend to ensure improvements? • What challenges are your practices experiencing with filling their schedules or meeting same-day access? • What are we doing to improve our access?
People	• What development opportunities are there for your leaders this week? • What are the current challenges with regard to staffing/coverage? • Human Resources challenges? • Who do we want to recognize/celebrate this week? • What provider issues do I need to aware of?
Cost	• How have we managed our overtime and labor expenses? • How is patient volume compared with budget expectations? What is driving any variance?
Wrap-up	• What are your priorities for this week? • What can I do to assist you this week? Items for me to follow up on:

observation visual by creating a regular schedule of what is to be observed, indicating what those tasks are and whether they were "red," out of compliance with the standard, or "green," in compliance with standard work.

Status Reports

Understanding the critical components of how the organization functions is vital for leaders. Status (what is referred to as Vitals Reports) reports are composed of a standard set of questions (**Table 1**) that covers the key operational and clinical priorities for the organization. Quality, safety, patient experience, finance, people, and environment are the domains reviewed at the beginning of each day by frontline leaders. These open-ended questions lead a structured conversation between leaders that ensures a deep understanding of business operations, promotes the development of critical thinking skills, helps to anticipate problems, and plans for the work of the day or week. The "Vitals Reports" cascade up the organizational chart, thereby aligning priorities top to bottom and creating a mechanism for escalation of issues in a timely manner.

Plan Do Study Act/Adjust

A key principle of Lean thinking is developing the capability to identify and solve problems at the frontline. This approach requires training the staff on a standard approach that guides them to develop and evaluate tests of change. A PDSA cycle (**Fig. 3**) is a

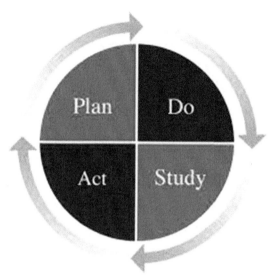

Fig. 3. PDSA cycle.

standard improvement methodology that codifies a scientific approach to problem solving, affords opportunity for learning for all parties involved, and ensures that proposed changes are making a positive impact. One of the defining features of PDSA is simplicity. It is designed to be an effective, yet easily understandable tool for frontline staff to engage change and create measureable improvement. The PDSA cycle consists of 4 distinct elements.

Plan
Before engaging in any activity, it is important to sufficiently plan for a test of change. Inadequate planning can lead to poorly designed interventions that waste time and financial resources. There are several key components in the planning stage, as follows:

- *Identify the team.* Tests of change can range from simple to complex, and it is important to ensure team members and their responsibilities are delineated. This delineation can include identification of a sponsor or champion depending on the activity's scale and scope.
- *Understand the problem.* It is important that all members of the team can agree on the answer to "What problem are we trying to solve?" As part of understanding the current state, the team should evaluate necessary data and/or observe relevant processes. Once the problem is clearly defined, root cause analysis is conducted to ensure the targeted improvement efforts are focused on the real causes and not symptoms.
- *Design the countermeasure.* Once the team has a firm grasp of the current state, it is important to plan the countermeasure to address the root cause or causes of the problem. Appropriate planning allows for clear understanding of activity scope while minimizing impact to ongoing operations.
- *Develop a data collection plan.* In advance, the team should decide what metrics will be needed to assess effectiveness, and how that data will be collected. Data collection need not be complex or sophisticated, but it is important that it be done thoughtfully.

Do

Once the "Plan" portion of a PDSA has been completed, the team can perform the countermeasure. Data collection is a requisite component of this activity.

Study

Once the "Do" portion of the PDSA cycle is underway, the team should evaluate its effectiveness. This evaluation should follow clearly from the current state assessment and the data collection plan that was previously developed. This step is critical to ensure any redesigned activity has been evaluated for effectiveness. This step is also a critical point of learning. Learning from countermeasures that did not yield the intended results can be just as valuable as learning from successes and can inform next steps.

Act/adjust

Based on the results of the evaluation, the team should reassess if their countermeasure has been effective, and what next steps will occur. If the intervention is successful, plans can be made to spread and sustain the new process across the organization. Alternatively, the team may choose to adjust the intervention and pursue a second PDSA cycle or design an entirely separate intervention.

In summary, PDSA is a simple yet powerful tool that helps guide frontline staff to effectively solve problems to root cause as a key component of their continuous improvement process.

Case Study, Continued

Betty Jo is beginning to make progress with the Hillandale Family Medicine team. After attending a training session during which she learned about creating a Daily Management System using Lean principles, she has instituted morning huddles to bring the team together before starting the clinic day. Currently, she is leading the huddle, but her nurse manager and practice medical director are both actively involved. They start by asking about any safety concerns and then move to an assessment of the "team mood" to make sure everyone is in a good place to engage in the work. A quick check-in then follows to review staffing for the day, capacity for same-day access, and any provider issues. The clinic is working on improving 2 of their quality metrics: blood pressure control and bundled metric for diabetes care, so efforts to improve those chosen measures are reviewed. Staff has suggested a couple of new ideas, and there is 1 ongoing PDSA test in the "work-in-process" section that is discussed. The huddle then closes with any staff celebrations or announcements, and everyone adjourns to begin their day. The process takes no more than 10 to 15 minutes, but helps to set the stage for the entire day. Betty Jo and her nurse manager then convene for their daily Vitals Report as part of their Leader Standard Work.

Lean Management

The authors believe the construct of "Align-Enable-Improve" creates the level of engagement and structure that connects daily work to achieving the overall strategic goals of the organization. This construct creates a framework that facilitates the spread of standard work, monitors and manages drift, supports the spread of continuous improvement, and promotes respect for people, including the leaders (**Box 3**). *Alignment* is critical to connect the frontline focus with upper-level leadership's priorities, all pointing toward the strategic goals (often referred to as *True North* goals) of the organization. Leaders can *enable* frontline problem solving and continuous improvement by demonstrating behaviors that support their staff through listening, coaching, and asking effective questions. *Improvement* happens through application

---

Box 3
Framework for management

Align the Important
• The strategic few

Improve the Process
• Systems in place

Enable the People
• People-centered culture

---

of A3 thinking (discussed later) and PDSA cycles that are grounded in the scientific method to solve problems.

A3 Thinking

A3 thinking (A3 paper size used in the metric system) is an approach to problem solving that starts with a clear problem statement and the context as to why solving this problem is important to the organization. It provides an understanding of the current state and outlines what the target state should look like. The A3 will highlight the gap between current and target state, possible root causes of the problem, and then propose countermeasures that could be tested to address these root causes. PDSA cycles can then be run as rapid cycle experiments to determine if these countermeasures actually solve the problem or need to be adjusted and tested again. Successful interventions are then implemented and spread across the organization. A3 thinking is grounded in the scientific method in that hypotheses are tested, data are collected, and only change that results in improvement is implemented.

It is important to keep in mind that A3 thinking is a dynamic process based on coaching and learning. Although achieving identified outcomes is important, the primary focus is on gaining a deeper understanding of the gap between current state and target state. It reflects how much is learned in the process of testing countermeasures and how lessons are taught to others. The roles of leaders are to demonstrate behaviors that encourage critical thinking and to coach problem-solving skills that focus on improving the process rather than achieving an outcome. Outcomes are achieved through process improvement, which then creates the opportunity to establish new targets.

The creation and utilization of an A3 are a dynamic process that functions as a guide for improvement work. The A3 is important in telling the story about a particular improvement effort and allows the history of countermeasures and adjustments to be captured.[7] Revisiting the A3 over time confirms that improvements are being sustained and opportunity is being created to test new countermeasures as the standard is changed and improved. PDSA cycles go hand in hand with creating and using A3 thinking as a tool to address problems. For example, one could develop an A3 to outline an overall approach to complex care management as part of the population health strategy. This approach would include a problem statement and background information along with a clear outline of the current state and desired target state. Countermeasures are then proposed and tested through multiple PDSA cycles that move the organization or clinic closer to the target state. Using the A3 tool also creates accountability by assigning responsibility for certain activities and asking the question "by whom, by when" as countermeasures are tested.

Leader Standard Work

Just as frontline staff has standard work that defines their daily processes, leaders can also develop standard work that reinforces the activities and behaviors needed to demonstrate their organizational commitment to continuous improvement. As David Mann[8] states in his book, *Creating a Lean Culture,* "Leader standard work provides a structure and a routine that helps leaders shift for a sole focus on results to a dual focus on process plus results." The goal of creating standard work for leaders is to help them move away from "firefighting" as a response to problems. The leader is then in a position to anticipate issues, have a line of sight to the *Gemba* (workplace where value is created), and provide opportunities for coaching and learning. It is important for leaders to create space in their calendars for these behaviors to happen, rather than layer them on top of an already busy schedule. Leader standard work consists of a series of activities and behaviors that keep the organization focused on solving problems that result in sustainable improvement. A medical assistant may have 95% of their work defined in a standard work document, whereas middle managers and senior leaders will have anywhere from 25% to 75% of their time outlined in standard work activities. Examples of what a senior leader may include in their standard work might include time spent in observation and coaching, regular purposeful Gemba walks, scheduled reviews of data and metrics, and scheduled time to prepare for meetings and presentations. Engaging in standard work supports the ideal that leaders should possess a deep understanding of the current state of their organization before they can develop strategies and implement tactics that move the organization forward. Rather than solving problems on their own, it puts them in a position to coach those who report to them on developing their own problem-solving skills and sustaining improvements that are aligned with the organizations goals.

Just as it is important for an organization to exhibit discipline in adherence to continuous improvement work, it is also important for leaders to remain disciplined in maintaining their standard work. One strategy the authors have found useful is for leaders to put their standard work document in a format that allows for documentation of completion of these activities on a weekly, monthly, or quarterly schedule. They also make these documents public, which creates a level of accountability to themselves and their colleagues.

Training Program

Training and developing leaders to this new way of thinking and behaving takes a multipronged approach. Knowledge of the tools and processes can be gained through classroom instruction, but true understanding can only come from doing the work. The authors' philosophy is to combine classroom teaching with on-the-job coaching to achieve the greatest adoption (**Table 2**).

The Foundations course includes a simulation exercise to introduce the concepts of process improvement and multiple, iterative PDSA cycles. The concepts of standard work, how to 5S a workplace (Sort, Set in order, Shine, Standardize, Sustain), and process mapping are covered in this course. The Advanced PDSA course introduces participants to A3 thinking along with understanding problem definition and root cause analysis. The curriculum also includes instruction in countermeasure development then leads into countermeasure development, the best use of data, and action planning to test proposed PDSA cycles.

The Leadership course introduces the concepts associated with the authors' Lean management system. This course is where participants discover the concepts of Gemba walks and how to develop and use their Leader Standard work. There is

Table 2
Training program example

	PreRequisite	Time	Training Topics
DPC Continuous Improvement Foundations	DPC Orientation (Introduction to CIS and PDSA)	6 h	Introduction to Lean principles and tools PDSA 8 Wastes 5 S Standard Work Process Mapping Continuous Flow How to use data for improvement
Advanced PDSA (A3) Thinking	Continuous Improvement Foundation Course, Lean Healthcare 225 (North Carolina State University) OR Lean Six Sigma Green Belt	Series: Part 1: 4-h workshop Part 2: 1:1 coaching session Part 3: 4-h workshop Part 4: 1:1 coaching session All parts of the series must be completed	PDSA (A3) Thinking Problem Identification Root Cause Analysis Using data to evaluate results Countermeasure Development Action Planning
Leading in a Culture of Continuous Improvement	CI Foundations Course Advanced PDSA Thinking	Part 1: 5 h *Coaching/Action Period* Part 2: 8 h *Coaching/Action Period* Part 3: 5 h	CIS 2.0 Gemba Walks Leader Standard Work Process Observation Visual Management Daily/weekly status reports Facilitating change management Prioritizing improvement efforts Coaching for improvement Improvement huddles

Abbreviations: CI, continuous improvement; CIS, continuous improvement system.

also discussion of how the authors' system of Daily management functions using the Continuous Improvement System along with process observation that happens in the practice environment. There is time to learn coaching skills and to role-play this activity with other class participants. The system of daily and weekly Status reports is also introduced in this session.

Case Study, Concluded

Betty Jo's morning commute is no longer filled with dread as she drives to the office. Her daily management system has the entire clinic engaged in problem-solving and improvement work, and her metrics have improved as a result. The clinic has yet to hit its quality targets, but the clinic leaders and staff have made significant improvements and have a plan that should achieve success within the next 3 months. Patients are happier as evidenced by their Global Rating score, and the staff call-outs and turnover have dramatically improved. The providers have noticed the improvements and are talking less about burnout and more about how engaged the staff is in working as a team. Through her weekly Vitals Reports with her Regional Administrator, Betty Jo is able to appropriately escalate issues and receive coaching on solving problems at her level. She now has time to focus on strategic efforts related to developing her teams, growing the practice, and implementing the new Behavioral Health program because the staff is engaged in solving the problems that had previously landed on her desk.

Spreading and sustaining

How best to spread and sustain Lean management is a challenging question that often causes organizations to struggle. It can be useful to start with problem-solving skills and spread these concepts across the system in an "inch-deep and mile-wide" approach. This method can help to create engagement and avoid the "project-of-the-month" mentality. The authors believe it is also useful to use the "model cell" approach, "mile-deep and inch-wide," to pilot and test interventions in a single unit or practice before spreading throughout the organization. This approach provides an opportunity for others to go and see how the work is done and can help with engagement when spread does begin to happen. It also provides a training site and can expose unanticipated workflow challenges. It will provide an environment that allows a deeper understanding of the current state and ensures the appropriate testing of countermeasures geared toward creating improvement.

Embedding processes and activities that maintain the spirit of continuous improvement can prevent the inevitable regression back into old habits. It will be important to maintain the discipline of supporting the daily management system and demonstrating leadership behaviors that are consistent with Lean Management. This way of thinking and behaving then becomes the new norm in the organization for solving problems, engaging in performance improvement, and strategic planning.

It is important to think of Lean transformation as a new way to manage the organization. This work should not be viewed as a project with a "beginning" and an "end," but as a continuous journey toward becoming a learning health system that delivers high value care. The principles of a Lean system, solving problems to root at the frontline, respect for people, avoiding waste and rework, relentless focus on process improvement, and leaders with humble listening skills and coaching behaviors, lend themselves well to success in improving population health through clinical care, where the focus is on creating value. Success in a population health approach requires organizations to focus on improving access, closing quality gaps in care, reducing cost and overutilization, and improving the patient experience. This work can benefit from the efficiencies and improvements gained through adoption of the principles, practices, and behaviors consistent with a Lean way of thinking and acting. Best of all, this can be a key component of returning joy to the work of the clinicians and staff.

REFERENCES

1. Mann D. Creating a lean culture. 3rd edition. CRC Press, Taylor and Francis Group. Florida 2014.
2. Available at: https://www.shingo.org/model. Accessed December 28, 2018.
3. Catalysis. Available at: https://createvalue.org/wp-content/uploads/Systems-Approach-for-Transforming-Healthcare-Organizations.pdf. Accessed December 28, 2018.
4. Rother M. Toyota Kata: managing people for improvement, adaptiveness and superior results. New York: McGraw-Hill; 2010. p. 39.
5. Liker J, Convis G. The Toyota way to lean leadership. New York: McGraw-Hill; 2012. p. 95.

6. Rother M. Toyota kata: managing people for improvement, adaptiveness, and superior results. New York: McGraw-Hill; 2010. p. 163.
7. Barnas K, Adams E. Beyond heroes: a lean management system for healthcare. ThedaCare Center for Healthcare Value; 2014. p. 69.
8. Mann D. Creating a Lean culture, tool to sustain lean conversions. 3rd edition. CRC Press; 2015. p. 51–74.

Tools for Population Health Management

Robert W. Fields, MD, MHA[a,b,*], Niyum Gandhi, BA[c]

KEYWORDS

- Population health • Tools for population health • Patient portals
- Provider engagement • Patient engagement • Data integration • Data visualization
- Analytics

KEY POINTS

- Data integration and visualization tools are key elements of population health management operations.
- Clinical operations require tools that can help segment the population into actionable cohorts, create care plans that can be shared among important stakeholders as well as provide the business intelligence needed to manage teams.
- Both provider and patient engagement tools are important as systems attempt to shift behavior and culture toward value.
- Engagement tools need to go beyond just education and supply insights at the appropriate times and in the right formats to affect change.

INTRODUCTION

For providers and those who deliver health care services, one of the more challenging aspects of population health management is that many delivery system workflows and technology tools, from those at the largest of academic health centers to solo practitioners, were largely built to optimize coding and billing and less for quality and outcomes. Such tools are helpful for maximizing volume, tracking appointments, listing diagnoses, and following outbound claims and other discrete information ideal for a fee-for-service environment, but they are less helpful in the more complex analyses required to ensure desired outcomes with low variation, high reliability, and safety. Because of this limitation, providers are faced with the need to include new tools, solutions, and workflows all designed to help value-based outcomes. Solutions and tools without a population health strategy, however, do not often lead to desired results. In

Disclosure Statement: The authors have nothing to disclose.
[a] SVP and CMO Population Health, Mount Sinai Health System, 1 Gustave Levy Place, Box 1475, New York, NY 10029, USA; [b] The Institute for Family Health; [c] Health System Design and Global Health, Mount Sinai Health System, 1 Gustave Levy Place, Box 1475, New York, NY 10029, USA
* Corresponding author. 1 Gustave Levy Place, Box 1475, New York, NY 10029.
E-mail address: robert.fields@mountsinai.org

Prim Care Clin Office Pract 46 (2019) 529–538
https://doi.org/10.1016/j.pop.2019.07.012
0095-4543/19/© 2019 Elsevier Inc. All rights reserved.

other words, new tools alone are not enough. We outline the general categories of tools available for population health management as well as possible use cases that can help guide strategy. For the purposes of this article, we divide population health management tools into the following categories: (1) data and analytics, (2) clinical operations (including performance management), (3) patient engagement, and (4) provider engagement.

DATA AND ANALYTICS

If population health is defined as the health outcomes of a group of individuals, including the distribution of such outcomes within the group,[1] then it stands to reason that robust data and analytics are required to understand how health care is consumed, financed, and accessed within the population. Effective population health management requires a full picture of where and when patients get care and the funds flows that accompany this utilization. The 2 central elements of data and analytics for population health are the integration of data from a variety of disparate sources (eg, provider electronic health record data [EHR], payer claims) and the visualization of the key findings of the data.

Data Integration

One of the challenges to effectively manage population health is lack of comprehensive data. Typically, providers have EHR data, which is deep (full clinical and administrative data) but narrow (only encounters that occur with that provider). In contrast, health plans typically have claims files, which are broad (all clinical encounters for the patient) but shallow (only administrative data with limited clinical information). Identifying a way to integrate these 2 sources of data is essential. Many times, provider organizations get paralyzed in pursuit of the perfect amalgamation of data, often searching for additional sources to refine their understanding. We recommend that providers start with what they have and then seek to bring in additional data where possible, keeping in mind that none of the data are useful unless actionable. That is, based on the data, can the system do something with, for, or to a patient differently? Taking action based on data increases the burden for integration into workflow as well.

Organizing integrated data is critical for population health management. Although the aim is to improve the health of the full population, data integration needs to happen at the level of the individual patient. When effectively integrated, the EHR provides a look at the clinical picture (eg, the patient has an elevated blood pressure) and claims files give insight into where the patient gets care (eg, the patient went to an out-of-town emergency department with elevated blood pressure). For an organization that is responsible for the health of the population the "spine" for population health efforts is the attribution file that lists all the patients in the population. Attribution files are notoriously error prone[2] but here we advocate for an approach in which "perfect should not be the enemy of the good." Organizations often include data from other sources including partner organizations, public use files, and other sources. Data integration at all levels needs to be in the context of the Health Insurance Portability and Accountability Act of 1996 and any other applicable privacy laws.[3]

Data storage

Storage of integrated data can be challenging. Among the challenges are cost, security, and fluidity of data. The examples that follow highlight some tools for storage. Our goal is not to advocate for a specific method among many, but to highlight the options and tradeoffs.

Centralized health information exchange

Per the mandate of Office of the National Coordinator for Health Information Technology, Regional Health Information Organizations and other forms of Health Information Exchanges (HIE) have been supported through a mix of public and private initiatives.[4] These organizations typically function as hub-and-spoke models, whereby all participating providers provide their data to the HIE that functions as a business associate for those participating providers to gather and integrate the data. Then, providers can pull these data down, either through data feeds or a portal the HIE has developed, when needed for a valid purpose. The advantages of this model are that the HIE can build services on top of the data rather easily to get actionable information to providers. Examples include clinical event notifications for admissions/discharges, missed medication notifications (if the HIE gets information from pharmacies as well), analytics on high-risk patients, and so forth. The disadvantage of this model is that it can be costly to maintain a centralized repository of the data and it can be challenging to manage a distributed governance model (deciding what capabilities to invest in) across all of the participants or customers of the HIE.

Proprietary health information exchanges or enterprise data warehouses

Some population health management organizations have built their own data repositories to pull these data from various sources. These data repositories can be on-premise data warehouses or cloud-based and can be standalone or feed into other systems (such as the EHR). The advantages of this model are the same as the HIE model, with the additional advantage of customization to a specific provider's needs.[5] The disadvantages are that the infrastructure costs are borne by just one provider and the privacy/consent model needs to be managed by that one provider as well. In addition, to the extent collaboration across a broad range of provider entities is needed to improve population health, this model can be more challenging to spread/scale.

Point-to-point data integration

Increasingly, through better standards development, the private EHR market is responding to provider needs by bringing lower cost options to market. Most notably, through Carequality[6] (governed by the Sequoia Project) and the CommonWell Alliance,[7] several large EHR vendors have collaborated to use a standards-based model for sharing data between providers directly through the EHR.[8] As this model expands to health plans and other vendors, it may present a more scalable national model for data integration and sharing. The advantages of this model are that it provides greater scalability across a broad range of providers, with little to no centralized infrastructure costs. It also, by definition, integrates data directly into the workflow. There are disadvantages, including that currently there are limited analytics and insights built in this model, because there is no central body pulling in the data that can build notifications, alerts, and other insights onto the integrated data. Another disadvantage is that a potentially more complicated/challenging consent framework that may limit the ability to share data without explicit consent versus what can be done with private/public HIEs for treatment purposes without consent. It is important to note that this is a rapidly emerging area, so its advantages/disadvantages are changing by the month. In reality, currently most effective population health managers are using a mix of all of these models to meet their needs, but as the industry advances, more dominant models for specific needs will likely emerge.

Data Visualization

As difficult as it can be to gather data from all the various entry points in complex systems, effective visualization of the data is critical to make the most of these efforts.

Visualization enables terabytes of data to be distilled into potentially actionable elements.

For physicians and other providers whose primary function is patient care, it is unlikely that they will view data in tools that are separate from the EHR. Unless compensation structures and schedules are adjusted to account for population health management activities outside of patient care, the best strategies for sharing and visualizing data include "just in time" data presentation related to the patients being seen that day or within a window of impact. Information such as inpatient or emergency room utilization, quality gaps, clinical pathways, and/or other relevant guidance can drive practice operations either via previsit planning or direct outreach when the patient arrives in the clinic or other health setting. In addition, panel-level reports such as risk-adjusted panel size, high-risk reports, or other similar descriptive data points can be helpful in the context of panel rounds with multidisciplinary teams within the health care setting. For example, developing and executing on plans of care for high-risk patients who are not in the clinic requires a tool that can quickly provide risk scores, cost and utilization information, and other relevant information necessary for appropriate outreach by the care team.

Care managers also require data visualization that can guide their work. At a minimum, data visualization tools, either as a standalone or ideally integrated into care management platform workflows, should help dictate which patients receive outreach, are offered enrollment into various care management programs, or receive other interventions. Similar to the clinic rounds described previously, important data points include cost and utilization data, risk stratification scores, and predictive analytics scores that help define the most appropriate populations for intervention.

Predictive analytics, population stratification, and other data tools

Risk stratification and predictive risk scores are often confused and misused in population health operations. Risk stratification scores are data elements that are descriptive in nature (not predictive of specific outcomes) and best used to compare individuals within a population for the purposes of prioritization or for risk adjusting populations.

Predictive risk scores tend to predict a specific outcome (eg, readmissions, new admissions, mortality, others) and therefore help direct a strategy that can include particular care management programs or interventions, office visits, or other types of outreach. Knowing the outcome determined by particular risk scores helps designers know where those scores should appear in the visualization and within the workflow of the person using the score. For example, a readmissions predictive score is certainly helpful for a care manager working on transitions of care but it is also helpful for providers seeing a patient in clinic after an index admission and even for the inpatient care managers working on discharge planning.

CLINICAL OPERATIONS
Care Management Documentation and Panel Management

Care managers, including nurses, social workers, care coordinators, and other disciplines, require tools to both manage their caseload and to document interactions and care plans to drive improved clinical and financial outcomes. Many EHR companies have designed associated care management platforms with the promise that increased integration with physician workflows will lead to improved operations. Although this integration is important, there are other factors to consider.

Managing a team of care managers requires an understanding of active caseloads to measure workload and productivity. Productivity can be measured as number of encounters, completion of tasks, or via other process metrics. Caseloads may be risk-adjusted so that the total volume of work remains equitable within the team. For the care manager, these tools often provide a summary of their current roster of patients, including information on pending tasks, a schedule of encounters for the day, alerts for new items, such as admissions or discharges, and other important information. Supervisors often have other views that evaluate the population as a whole with metrics on utilization cost, risk, and other summary information and either role should easily be able to run reports on current caseloads, pending tasks, number of encounters, and other relevant data.

Assessments are generally the first important workflow element within the platform and can be specified to the program being considered. Regardless of the type of assessment, the most advanced tools include branching logic such that individual responses can lead to more in-depth questions where necessary and guide the care manager in gathering the most appropriate information. Automation can be helpful by creating care plan elements based on assessment responses.

Care plans are a critical element of any care management platform. In many cases, care management platforms allow for sharing of the care plan with the patients or family members via paper, e-mail, portal, or other methods. More advanced tools also allow for sharing of care plans within the community such that hospitals, emergency rooms, physician offices, and even nonprofits working on social determinants can meaningfully engage in the care plan and complete tasks.

Combining data, analytics, and operations

Operational effectiveness in population health management requires bringing data and analytics to operations in a useable, actionable form. Integration of admission/discharge/transfer feeds from various hospitals into the care management platform may drive the work of a transitions care manager without having to use an outside platform. The addition of risk stratification scores can help prioritize lists of patients by those who are at highest risk or are most likely to benefit from the work of the individual care manager. Predictive analytics integration can also define specific care management programs, and knowing those scores can provide important context for the care manager as they interact with patients. The most sophisticated tools include data from EHRs and claims such as medication lists and utilization histories, emergency room and inpatient utilization over time, associated physician providers, and, in some cases, social determinants information gathered from various sources.[9] All of these data elements help to not only define and prioritize the work but also provide important context in discussion with the patient.

PATIENT AND PROVIDER ENGAGEMENT
Patient Engagement

Engaging patients/consumers in their health is critical to population health. The Healthcare Information and Management Systems Society provides a framework that can help us think about the necessary tools.[10]

Information/transparency

Over the past few years, there has been a proliferation of transparency tools designed to give the patient more information from wayfinding and physician directories to transparency across quality, patient satisfaction, and costs.[11] Given the population health goals of achieving the Triple Aim, giving patients access to transparent information that helps them select providers/services can be an important lever in ensuring delivery of high-value care. In the absence of vetted transparency, patients will rely on unvalidated transparency, so it is important that these types of data are meaningful and actionable to help patients make appropriate decisions for their care. These data include patient satisfaction data. The University of Utah made waves when they became the first academic medical center to post online patient satisfaction scores of their own physicians with a 5-star rating system and patient comments in December 2012.[12] Since then, many others have followed, using this strategy as a key way to improve patient satisfaction and engage patients with transparent information.

Given how much cost patients now bear for their own health care, transparency regarding cost estimation is also important. It is now possible to integrate cost information with eligibility verification to give real-time information at a patient-specific level based on their benefits.

E-visits/e-tools/forms

Population health management is intended to move us from reactive, break/fix care to proactive prevention. Population health managers need to meet the patients where they are and want to be, not necessarily requiring an in-person visit for all care. In addition, with patients increasingly behaving as consumers, they want to interact with providers and care teams on their own terms not on ours, even for episodic care.[13] To adapt to changing delivery expectations, systems require both clinical and administrative tools. Although this effort can start with simple native tools, such as secure messaging, increasingly even more sophisticated solutions are available in the EHR such as e-visits and interactive care plan management. Ideally, these activities, currently tied to in-person visits, would increasingly move to virtual as population health managers take on responsibility for total cost of care and fee-for-service billing becomes less important. They are both more efficient (and therefore less costly) done virtually, and more convenient for the patient (promoting adherence).

In a more advanced way, remote monitoring helps move to true proactivity and can be either disease-focused (eg, glucose, weight, electrocardiogram) or more wellness-focused (eg, physical activity tracking, nutrition guidance). It is important to note with all of these that the technology is often the simple part, culture change and operations are needed to really make this work. Engaging patients offline through other platforms requires the right operations to actually be useful. For example, there is no value in tracking weight for patients with heart failure through wireless scales if no one intervenes when it falls out of range. There is no value in having telemedicine available technically if clinicians do not structure their practice workflow in a way in which they can use it.

Consumers are now expecting the same level of ease in health care as they do in other industries, such as airlines (book online, check-in online), ride-sharing applications (request a ride, pay seamlessly), and e-commerce (get recommendations, shop easily, have things delivered to the door).[14] "Administrative" tools make the consumer experience easier with the hope of increasing appropriate care (and modes of care delivery) and improving outcomes. These tools include online scheduling, online forms management, online bill pay, and online prescription refill requests. All of these also have the added benefit of reducing operating cost for providers if done well. Similar to clinical tools, operations are often harder to implement than the technology. Online scheduling technology is easy; standardizing visit types and ensuring clinicians are comfortable opening up their schedules is harder.

Patient access and use (including interoperability and collaborative care)

Patient access starts with something as simple as giving the patient access to the medical record, but it is critical to expand this access to include as much of the integrated clinical record as possible. This expanded access can include laboratory results and prescriptions, as well as inputs from other settings of care using the data exchange and integration tools mentioned earlier in the article. More sophisticated organizations allow patients to share this access easily with other care teams and with caregivers or family members. Going further, some organizations are now allowing patient-selected applications to interact with these data, truly putting patients in control of their data.[15] This tactic has become increasingly possible because of the work of the Argonaut Project, a private-sector initiative supported by the major EHR vendors to use a standards-based approach based on the Fast Healthcare Interoperability Resources application programming interface framework to allow for these types of integrations on a scalable manner.[16]

Patient-specific education

Once we have met the patients' most pressing online needs (book care, receive care, pay for care, access their health information), we earn more of the right to engage them on the things necessary to manage care. We can start with simple education packages at the episodic or disease level that can be easily accessed. One example would be giving easy access to health information on general conditions that the physicians in the network have approved. This approach can expand to push capabilities by which clinicians "prescribe" the right educational modules; for example, a patient with diabetes is prescribed a diabetes education module. The most sophisticated approaches use algorithm-derived "push" information whereby information is triggered and delivered at specified times in response to a particular input. One example would be educational bits on diabetes pushed at the right points in time when the patient is already thinking about his diabetes (for example, by linking it to a diabetes remote monitoring solution and pushing the information right after the patient measures his or her blood glucose level).

Patient-generated data

Increasingly, the definition of the health record is expanding to include patient-generated data to improve care. Specifically, patient-reported outcome measures (PROMs), measurement instruments that patients complete to provide information on their health status, are increasingly being used as a complementary data source to traditional clinical measures.[17] Many PROM instruments have now been validated in the clinical setting, from generic tools that are applied across broad populations to condition-specific ones that relate to particular diseases or episodes of care.

We close this section with a note on patient portals. There is much discussion about the value of patient portals. It is important to think about portals from the patient perspective, not from the tool perspective. It is less about "having a patient portal" and more about making access to all of the preceding tools simple, seamless, and integrated. Ideally, there would be one easy place to get all of this information, and it would all be integrated whether the patient is pulling something down from a portal or application or whether the care team is pushing something to the patient via an alert or notification. Many EHR-based patient portals are configured such that they are modular enough to build all of this in. Some organizations choose to instead build or buy their own version that is EHR-agnostic and pull in the relevant functionality. This decision is an important one with high switching costs, but it is important to remember that for population health management success, it is less about the specific platform and more about the ease and integration of access to all of this information from the patient perspective.

Provider Engagement

Online portals are the primary way that network managers interact and share information with providers. Portals serve as a repository for network documents and agreements, compliance documents, required education, and quality performance. They can also have integrated data visualization elements such that a provider can easily see his or her performance along measures of utilization and quality. As a single source of truth for relevant documents, performance metrics and targets as well as other necessary information, provider portals are essential in the management of any population health network. However, it is our collective experience that relatively few providers in networks meaningfully engage in such portals, particularly during the early development of a network. Given the amount of time spent between e-mails and the EHR, management must either provide significant incentives to log on to the platform, or at a minimum a compelling call to action (eg, information on compensation). Although some networks have mandated logging on the portal a number of times per year, it is less clear how often that leads to an effective exchange of information. Personal exchanges with staff members from the network where performance information is discussed and shared can be an excellent supplement while also creating an opportunity for education with regard to portal use.

As more and more individuals use smartphones, phone applications can be used as a portal while simultaneously creating a means for communicating to care management at the point of care, monitoring performance or even participating in educational events via audio or video. Smartphone applications are portable and therefore can create enhanced opportunities to engage with the network. Creating continuing medical education or other educational opportunities and linking them with clinical programs or other clinical goals of the network remains a vital element of provider engagement and can often be administered via online portal or smartphone application.

Two other tools to consider are referral management systems and customer management systems. Referrals within the network are often a tracked metric for value-based networks. Given the goals of improved quality and lower cost (ie, improved value), it makes sense that providers within the network should keep their referrals within the network. Operationally, this can be difficult for a whole host of reasons, including long-standing professional relationships, geographic patterns, variations in quality, and other factors. Given that referral processes are highly variable within clinical points of care, tools that can either facilitate the referral process itself or gather and assimilate referral data can be a very important part of the strategy. Implementation of these tools can be as complete as having all referrals flow through the system to less robust integration where preferred providers are simply listed by region and specialty. Given increased energy around closing of referral loops and communication between primary care and specialty providers, however, more robust strategies (and tools) are often necessary.

Customer management systems help coordinate outreach to various providers in the network to avoid duplication of effort and perhaps frustration among network providers by having a system of outreach activities that can be referenced centrally. These tools are often used in customer-service environments and perform a similar function that often becomes necessary as networks grow and the number of stake-holders also grows.

SUMMARY

Population health management entities have the difficult task of fundamentally changing the relationships of patients to providers and systems, as well as those of providers to payers, hospitals, and other important partners in health care. Although it is obvious that even the best tools do not guarantee success in population health management, the wrong tools can absolutely sabotage best efforts. Therefore, thoughtful vetting of potential vendors and inclusion of relevant stakeholders during the selection process are important. In addition, keep in mind that the simplest solutions, even a paper report, can be very effective if designed appropriately and if the appropriate context is given. Last, proper management of the suite of solutions requires constructive partnerships with information technology and data teams at the institutional level. These tools require interconnectivity and integration to work well and the interdependency with these other important stakeholders in the institution demonstrate the idea that population health management is not just a system program but a radical change in the way we deliver health care.

REFERENCES

1. Kindig D, Stoddart G. What is population health? Am J Public Health 2003;93: 380–3.
2. Gourevitch MN, Cannell T, Boufford JI, et al. The challenge of attribution: responsibility for population health in the context of accountable care. Am J Public Health 2012;102:S322–4.
3. Vayena E, Dzenowagis J, Brownstein JS, et al. Policy implications of big data in the health sector. Bull World Health Organ 2017;96:66–8.
4. Office of the National Coordinator for Health Information Technology. US Department of Health and Human Services. Available at: https://web.archive.org/web/20081221170404/http://www.os.dhhs.gov/healthit/executivesummary.html. Accessed April 20, 2019.
5. Perna G. Interoperability & HIE: public vs. private HIEs (Part 1). Available at: https://www.hcinnovationgroup.com/interoperability-hie/article/13024098/public-vs-private-hies-part-1. Accessed April 25, 2019.
6. Carequality. What we do - carequality. Available at: https://carequality.org/what-we-do/. Accessed April 24, 2019.
7. CommonWell Health Alliance. Home - CommonWell Health Alliance. Available at: https://www.commonwellalliance.org. Accessed April 24, 2019.
8. CommonWell Health Alliance. Carequality and CommonWoll Health Alliance agree on connectivity and collaboration to advance interoperability - CommonWell Health Alliance. Available at: https://www.commonwellalliance.org/news-center/commonwell-news/carequality-commonwell-health-alliance-collaboration/. Accessed April 24, 2019.
9. Bates DW, Saria S, Ohno-Machado L, et al. Big data in health care: using analytics to identify and manage high-risk and high-cost patients. Health Aff 2014; 33:1123–31.
10. HIMSS. HIMSS patient engagement framework. Available at: https://www.himss.org/himss-patient-engagement-framework. Accessed April 24, 2019.
11. Durand D. The health care value transparency movement and its implications for radiology. J Am Coll Radiol 2015;12:51–8.

12. Miller T, Mulvihill S. Sharing information to help patients make decisions. Available at: https://uofuhealth.utah.edu/newsroom/news/2012/e-surveys-patient-satisfaction.php. Accessed April 28, 2019.

13. Advisory Board. 31915_MIC_Consumer_Growth_Study_WEB. Available at: https://www.advisory.com/research/market-innovation-center/studies/2016/-/media/778A7724187E445FA37FEB2E7331BBEA.ashx. Accessed 24 Apr. 2019.

14. Postelnicu L. Patients acting as consumers, demanding more ease, better tools. Available at: https://www.mobihealthnews.com/content/patients-acting-consumers-demanding-more-ease-better-tools. Accessed April 28, 2019.

15. Rosenberg J. Majority of hospitals allow patient access to health data; physicians, consumers want more digital interaction. Available at: https://www.ajmc.com/focus-of-the-week/majority-of-hospitals-allow-patient-access-to-health-data-physicians-consumers-want-more-digital-interaction. Accessed April 24, 2019.

16. 2.14.1 The Argonaut Project. FHIR 2nd DSTU Draft For Comment. Available at: https://www.hl7.org/implement/standards/fhir/2015Jan/argonauts.html. Accessed April 24, 2019.

17. Wagle N. Implementing Patient-Reported Outcome Measures (PROMs). Available at: https://catalyst.nejm.org/implementing-proms-patient-reported-outcome-measures/. Accessed April 24, 2019.

Patient Engagement

Narayana S. Murali, MD, Dip. NB, CPE[a],*, Craig E. Deao, MHA[b]

KEYWORDS

- Patient engagement • Patient activation • Compassion • Trust

KEY POINTS

- Patient engagement is emerging as a novel and important measure, distinct from patient satisfaction and patient experience.
- As health systems focus on population health, patient engagement will become increasingly important owing to its effect on both quality and costs.
- Caregivers can support patient engagement, especially through evidence-based communication practices that demonstrate compassion and build trusting relationships.

INTRODUCTION

Improving population health requires improving the health of individual people, each of whom has different abilities and willingness to improve her own health. Patient engagement is highly predictive of both quality outcomes and health systems costs, the twin objectives under value-based health care efforts. Therefore, how engaged a person is in managing his or her health is a critical metric both to understand and to shape in the pursuit of improving population health.

DEFINING PATIENT ENGAGEMENT

You cannot enter any world for which you do not have the language.
—*Wittgenstein*

Although there is no widely accepted definition of patient engagement, the concept is that patients are actively involved in their health—in terms of processing information, deciding how care fits in their lives, and acting on those decisions.[1]

Engaged patients strive to be informed about their health, are involved in health care decisions, and participate in self-care. They assume responsibility and accountability for the role their behaviors play in their care outcomes. They self-monitor and provide information; they offer feedback on their experience and outcomes and commit to

Disclosure Statement: The authors have nothing to disclose.
[a] Marshfield Clinic Health System, Marshfield Clinic, Suite 1J2, 1000 North Oak Avenue, Marshfield, WI 54449, USA; [b] Studer Group, 350 West Cedar Street, Suite 300, Pensacola, FL 32502, USA
* Corresponding author.
E-mail address: Murali.Narayana@marshfieldclinic.org

making long-term lifestyle changes. They take greater responsibility for their health, which may be the single biggest lever we have for improving outcomes and decreasing costs in health care today.[2]

One of the most widely used instruments to assess this concept is the Patient Activation Measure—or PAM scale—that assesses patients based on 10 (or 13) questions about their personal experience, skills, knowledge, and commitment to make lifestyle changes. Increasingly in use across the health care system, in June 2016 the National Quality Forum endorsed this measure as a patient- and family-centered care measure.[3] It is also supported by the National Committee for Quality Assurance and has been adopted by National Health Service England for system-wide use within clinics, hospitals, and social services.

Hibbard defines patient activation as "the patient's knowledge, skills, ability, and willingness to manage his own health and care" and assigns "four distinct activation levels with specific needs, goals, and approaches to move the patient toward self-directed management."[4] Hibbard's patient activation assessments ask patients their level of agreement or disagreement with certain statements (ie, "I am confident I can tell a doctor my concerns, even when he or she does not ask," or, "I know what each of my prescribed medications does").

Based on their responses, patients are scored on a 0 to 100 scale. The score can be used to sort patients into 4 categories or "levels of activation," where the lowest level (level 1) describes a patient with a very passive approach to his health care, and the highest level (level 4) describes a patient with a proactive approach to partnering in health care. As a result, PAM scores represent an important and foundational tool to assess patient readiness for engagement.

"When it comes to activation, it's about supporting a patient's skill development and competence," explains Hibbard. "The goal is to create an environment so that patients can do for themselves because we've helped them acquire the skills they need to succeed." In other words, engagement is not some type of intervention with a patient.

Just as we know from our own life experience that we cannot change anyone, we also cannot make patients become activated. We can only make the conditions ripe for activation. That is, we can create an environment that supports others' ability and willingness to change.

To effectively support population health, health care systems need to create an environment in which the health-promoting choice is the easiest choice. It is very similar to the idea behind the use of defaults, such as autoenrollment in a company 401(k) plan. If we enroll employees automatically in the plan, but allow them to opt out, more employees will grow their savings by default.

There are multiple examples of using defaults in health care today. In 1 study, researchers found that long-acting but reversible methods of contraception were almost 22% more effective than refillable methods, like birth control pills and patches.[5] Why? It is easy, convenient, and likely to continue once the initial decision has been made, much like the 401(k) automatic enrollment scenario.

Within the context of population health, patient engagement (or activation) provides a novel understanding of how likely a patient will take ownership for his or her own health. The measure is particularly useful in care planning, providing much more usefulness than understanding only socioeconomic status, health literacy, or other social determinates of health. Those with lower levels of activation can be assigned additional supportive resources, whereas those with higher levels of activation would require less. For example, 1 organization uses PAM scores to tailor care pathways for patients with back pain by pairing a pain acuity score with the PAM so that high scorers on both measures might visit a physical therapist once a week to learn exercises and low scorers might visit 3 times per week for more support.[6] Using measures of patient engagement as part of the care planning process will facilitate the allocation of health system resources to optimize population health and effectively steward limited health system resources.

THE RISE OF THE CONCEPT OF PATIENT ENGAGEMENT

Patient engagement is a relatively new measure in the health care community. Just 20 years ago, the predominant patient-specific measures were indicators of their satisfaction with the health care they received. Always a critical measure for improving market share and identifying process improvement opportunities, these patient satisfaction surveys provide health systems with retrospective ratings from a group of patients focused on the factors associated with higher levels of service.

More recently, an additional set of measures has been added to provide additional insights into care quality as experienced by patients. The Consumer Assessment of Healthcare Providers and Systems (CAHPS) series of surveys have been a cornerstone of the Centers for Medicare and Medicaid Services' efforts to direct resources and patients toward higher value-producing health care providers. Although many health care practitioners conflate these CAHPS instruments with patient satisfaction instruments, their aims and methodology are quite distinct. Rather than asking patients to what degree they were satisfied with services received, the CAHPS measures ask patients to rate how frequently (never, sometimes, usually, or always) they observed specific practices occur while receiving health care, which are both observable by the patient and correlated with evidence-based care practices. As examples, rather than asking about whether the patient was highly satisfied with a particular aspect of their care, they are asked how often nurses explained things in a way they could understand; before giving them any new medicine, how often hospital staff described possible side effects in a way they could understand; and when they left the hospital, did they have a good understanding of the things they were responsible for in managing their health. Analyses of CAHPS results show strong correlations between patient ratings of these observable practices and traditional process of care and outcome measures of quality.

Both patient satisfaction and patient experience surveys (such as CAHPS) are of significant value to improve system results. These are both critical inputs for systemic efforts to improve quality, safety, and service, providing the voice of the customer into both defining and identifying opportunities for improving system results. However, because they are retrospective and reviewed at a group level, they provide few insights that help to improve health for specific individuals as they go through their unique care experiences.

The confusion around patient satisfaction and experience surveys stems from a lack of precision in the underlying items being measured. Ratings of customer satisfaction are distinct from ratings of how frequently a customer observed specific actions occurring around them. And these are equally distinct from measures of engagement.

Satisfaction is a measure of how well a person's expectations are being met. The customer is evaluating what they are receiving from the other party. Engagement, in general terms, is quite the opposite. Engagement is a customer's assessment of themselves—and the likelihood they will give discretionary effort or take ownership for their responsibilities.

A workplace example helps to clarify the distinction. An employee may be highly satisfied when their supervisor grants their request to leave work early on a particular day. However, that employee is unlikely giving discretionary effort to help advance that organization's mission in the time off work. Simply put, a person can experience high satisfaction and exhibit low engagement at the same time. Clearly, they are quite distinct. Numerous health care examples illustrate this contrast. As a classic example, a patient might be highly satisfied because he was prescribed an antibiotic; however, he may still not take that antibiotic.

Patient engagement measures, such as PAM scores, provide prospective, individual feedback that can help to shape the care provided to each patient based on their ability and willingness to manage their own health care. These attributes significantly increase the usefulness of patient engagement as a measure vital to improving population health, which requires patients to take an active role in such activities as changing lifestyle habits, participating in ongoing care modalities, and appropriately taking prescribed medications.

The evolution of patient engagement corresponds with the changing viewpoints within health care of the role patients play within the system, shifting from a paternalistic relationship to a partnership. No longer is the relationship described as what is done to" the patient or "for" the patient, but increasing "with" the patient.

With this shift comes a change in language. Although the term "patient" is widely used when a person is using the health care system, there is increasing recognition of the importance of the health care system to support health even when the person is not actively using traditional health care services. As a result, many health care organizations are introducing words such as consumer and customer to intentionally widen the aperture through which they view their end users.

Viewing patients through the broader lens as consumers invites consideration of how emerging disciplines such as behavioral economics can be used to support engagement, which we discuss in the section examining contemporary approaches to supporting patient engagement.

CURRENT STATE OF PATIENT ENGAGEMENT

The impact of patient engagement, or lack thereof, is profound within the context of population health. Approximately 40% of deaths are caused by modifiable behavioral issues.[7] Yet people with chronic diseases take only 50% of prescribed doses, 50% of patients follow referral advice, and 75% of patients do not keep their follow-up appointments.[7]

One of the most studied areas reflecting the importance of patient engagement in managing health is medication nonadherence, or the failure to take medications as prescribed. The reasons behind nonadherence are complex and multifactorial. To illustrate the magnitude of this challenge, in one 2008 study, more than 3% of prescriptions filled by the pharmacist were never picked up by the patient.[8] If this so-called prescription abandonment rate holds true for the 3.6 billion prescriptions filled in pharmacies that year, it means that 110 million prescriptions were abandoned in 2008. Of course, this number does not include the large percentage of patients who begin to take a prescription and discontinue it prematurely (eg, such as not completing an antibiotic course).

The positive effects of patient engagement on health care outcomes are compelling. The effects on reducing health care costs are equally striking. Chronic diseases, like cardiovascular diseases and diabetes, account for most deaths and more than 75% of the nation's medical care costs.[9] PAM scores are showing a clear link between patient activation and costs. Patients with the lowest activation have the most expensive costs, and vice versa.[10] As health systems look to understand and manage their true, unit costs as part of taking on financial risk within population health strategies, it will be critical to prospectively identify the individuals who will be associated with the greatest expenses so that resources can be allocated in support of their health and appropriate use of services.

Examining the causal factors that contribute to this association between patient activation and costs, highly engaged patients are more likely to perform the kinds of health-improving behaviors that correlate with better outcomes and lower long-term costs. As examples, highly engaged patients gain better control of high-density lipoprotein cholesterol and triglycerides, are less likely to smoke or be obese, are more likely to get pap smears and mammograms, have their depression controlled more appropriately, and have fewer emergency department visits and hospitalizations.[10]

SUPPORTING PATIENT ENGAGEMENT

The health care system and individual caregivers both have critical roles in supporting patient engagement. Central to implementing workable solutions is acknowledging the limitations that are perceived to be obstacles. For health systems, any strategy must be balanced against the myriad of competing options each vying for a limited set of financial resources. For individual caregivers, common obstacles include the perception that there is not enough time to support patient engagement, the extent to which patient engagement is seen as a meaningful dimension of population health, and the knowledge of strategies that can support patient engagement.

As systems consider their population health strategies, significant investments will be made in support of engagement, including patient portals, home monitoring, and patient education and behavior change tools. These resources can be significant to support patient knowledge, skills, abilities, and willingness to own their own health. A deeper discussion of these resources is covered in Robert W. Fields and Niyum Gandhi's article, "Tools for Population Health Management," in this issue.

Additionally, the decades-long efforts to organize care around patients rather than clinicians will yield greater convenience and access, further supporting patient engagement. As health care systems embrace the language of consumerism, behavioral economics can provide powerful insights to redesign care in ways that support engagement.

Behavioral economics updates the views of classical economics by injecting psychological insights that illuminate why people act in seemingly irrational ways. This insight can be especially helpful to understand many of the underlying challenges health care system leaders face as they seek to improve population health. For example, the book "Irrationality in Health Care"[11] sheds insight on such questions as:

- Why are behaviors detrimental to health, such as smoking and poor nutritional choices, hard to stop while behaviors that support health, such as exercise, hard to start?
- Why do patients sometimes not take the medicines they are prescribed?
- How can the explanation of risks and benefits influence whether a patient decides to undergo a particular procedure?

Although the underlying theories that explain these challenges are enlightening, much more exciting are the ideas this discipline offers for how we can address them. As an example, the use of commitment devices can be powerful in helping individuals commit to making health-promoting changes such as smoking cessation or adhering to an exercise regimen. To experience this for yourself, consider creating a contract on the www.stickK.com website.

In an effort to lose weight, Dean Karlan, a Professor of Behavioral Economics at Yale University, experienced the power of commitment contracts, which encourage people to achieve goals by leveraging concepts such as loss aversion. He and his cofounders developed this online goal setting tool to make this approach accessible.

To use the tool an individual selects a goal, a support group that can cheer on progress, a referee who assesses compliance, and what the individual would forfeit if unsuccessful. The latter category offers some ingenious options, including payments made to "anti-charities" when goal milestones are missed. For example, users in the UK can select from several football clubs. Some people might just exercise if the penalty for failing to do so is boosting their most despised team!

How could a health system leverage examples such as StickK to support patient engagement? Given the significant investment already made in connecting patients to the health system digitally, many health systems already have much of the infrastructure in place to incorporate similar approaches.

In addition to these system strategies, there are many practical and low-cost solutions caregivers can use immediately that can have significant influence on patient engagement. In selecting approaches for implementation, there most be recognition that caregivers already feel they have too much to do in too little time with each patient. What can be done that has the maximal impact on engagement in the shortest amount of time?

A resource on this topic is the book, "Compassionomics: The Revolutionary Scientific Evidence that Caring Makes a Difference."[12] Covering the findings of more than 1000 scientific abstracts and 200 research papers, the book concisely summarizes the evidence that compassion—the emotional response to another's pain or suffering, involving an authentic desire to help—has a clear impact on both quality and cost, the twin aims of value-based population health care.

The book reviews the evidence supporting the link between caregiver compassion and patient activation, patient engagement, and patient enablement. Research shows that compassionate patient care is associated with better patient activation and engagement and, as a result, better patient self-care. Physician compassion can drive patients to be more engaged in their health care and to want to have more information on both treatment options and health promotion, which is associated with better long-term outcomes and enhanced quality of life.

One study of patients with diabetes found significantly greater adherence to medications with better interpersonal connection, specifically when patients had more trust in the health care provider. Perhaps this finding explains, at least to some extent, why research has found that health care provider compassion is associated with better blood glucose control and fewer complications requiring hospitalization among patients with diabetes.

Patient engagement can be supported by trust, the relationship a patient has with their providers. Even simple acts can significantly build trust. When clinicians sit with a patient rather than stand, it flattens the authority gradient between those who give care and those who receive it. Flat authority gradients yield better communications: patients are more likely to share pertinent information, as an example. Additionally, although sitting takes no more time than standing, the literature shows that it increases the perception of time spent with the patient by about 50%.[13]

For years, much of the work on engaging patients in safety practices has centered on asking them to speak up if something does not seem right. Such a strategy may not be effective. One study aimed at improving patient safety and reducing medical errors showed that many patients are uncomfortable asking their clinician even basic questions like, "How long will I be in the hospital?"[14] When considering more challenging questions like, "I don't think that is the medication I am on. Can you check please?" or "Have you washed your hands?", patients were very unlikely to speak up. Given that patient safety requires full engagement, patients must feel they can ask questions they perceive as challenging without offending their clinician.[14]

A second study on patient perceptions of safety in the hospital found that practices that we may consider routine in the health care setting are new to the patient.[15] However, it turns out that if we engage the patient in even a brief interaction—asking the patient to say her name aloud while the nurse reads the name on the label, for example—it can return an important sense of control to the patient.

THE MARSHFIELD CLINIC HEALTH SYSTEM EXPERIENCE WITH PATIENT ENGAGEMENT

The Marshfield Clinic Health System is one of the nation's premier rural, not-for-profit, fully integrated health care systems with more than 55 clinical locations, 6 hospitals, a research institute, a regional academic center, and the sixth largest health plan in the state of Wisconsin. The organization has served patients and consumers since 1916, with more than 1200 providers across 86 specialties, and more than 10,000 employees providing care to 34 Wisconsin communities with approximately 3.5 million patient encounters annually.

Like most other leading health care organizations, the Marshfield Clinic Health System has used traditional modalities such as patient portals, telehealth, and care coordinators, and relied on proprietary patient experience, quality outcome, or CAPHS surveys as proxy measures for patient engagement. On the health plan end, to enhance engagement, patients identified as having high-risk conditions or chronic diseases are managed by active outreach programs and nurse coordinators, while using net promoter scores as a measurement of engagement. The success of many of these discrete processes have at best been variable. Although patient portals, outreach calls from a health plan nurse, and technology may assist the motivated patients, they are inadequate in activating those patients who need high touch, resources, and support.

If a patient is ill and choses to seek medical care, engagement is assumed. Activation, in contrast, depends on the environment that supports it in addition to personal motivation. The former is determined, in no small measure, by the social determinants of health (income, education, employment, working conditions, housing, access to food, and social inclusion/exclusion). Beyond providing access to medical care, communities and proactive health systems should collaborate to address social determinants that influence health outcomes as well.

Over the past few years, we have piloted care models integrating the clinical provider team delivery and the health plan systematically coordinating resources and business analytics to engender active engagement thus enhancing the environment to achieve activation. The Heart Failure Improvement Clinic and the Hospital at Home are 2 such projects that operate on similar frameworks.

The Heart Failure Improvement Clinic, which has more than 1000 patients, generated the following outcomes per 100 patients when compared with their nonenrolled comparison group with similar disease state and comorbidities: a 15.6% decrease in emergency room use, a 11.6% decrease in hospital admission, and a 4.8% decrease in all-cause 30-day readmission. Importantly, the data revealed a 41.8% decrease in all-cause mortality. In a single point analysis of the 2016 cohort of 600 patients, using a risk-adjusted, 12-month cumulative spread method, we calculated $2.7 million in savings. There was a 2.9% increase in medical and treatment costs for patients who were eligible but not enrolled, compared with a 3.4% decrease in costs for the enrolled patients.

The Hospital at Home program, rechristened the Home Recovery Care Program, is a modernized approach to managing acutely ill patients at home in a 40-mile radius with a care transition team of hospitalists, home nursing, social workers, care coordinators, and ancillary staff while leveraging virtual health. In the past year, the Marshfield Clinic Health System provided such care for more than 250 patients, and is expanding this program to other sites. These are patients who traditionally would be admitted and managed on the med-surg floor of a hospital. Patients who came into the emergency room, chose care at home with an 88% conversion rate and a subsequent 95% top box response in patient satisfaction. Patients also experienced a 34% decrease in mean length of stay and 58% decrease in hospital readmissions.

In both models, the overarching framework involves proactive, early high-touch, engagement coupled with appropriate evidence based care pathways with ongoing regular follow-up. Education, counseling with motivational interviewing techniques, and lifestyle management are tailored to meet patient needs. A high-touch care team on the front end flattens the power differential between the caregivers and the recipients, enhances access, provides opportunity to understand and address the social determinants that affect engagement and activation while engendering increasing trust. To bridge vast distances in a rural environment, we harness readily available technology such as telehealth, remote monitoring, oral and intravenous medication management, and 24/7 nurse online support or home nursing care with physician oversight during the acute illness. A seamless link to our electronic medical records ensures care coordination, and information transparency. Both models focus on the patient, distinguish them as consumers who have a choice of where and how they seek care, and work with them to actively engage, motivate, and augment patient activation. These models have inherent costs that can be offset by shared savings, usually retained by the payer or the health plan. A partnership of the willing payer, a compassionate provider in an environment supportive of patient activation, and a motivated patient ultimately provide superior outcomes and lower total cost of health care.

REFERENCES

1. Gruman J, Rovner MH, French ME, et al. From patient education to patient engagement: implications for the field of patient education. Patient Educ Couns 2010;78(3):350–6. Available at: https://doi.org/10.1016/j.pec.2010.02.002. Accessed July 13, 2016.
2. Deao C. The E-factor: how engaged patients, clinicians, leaders, and employees will transform healthcare. Pensacola (FL): Firestarter Publishing; 2016.
3. PRWeb. Insignia health earns 'Best in Class' endorsement from National Quality Forum for a person and family-centered care measure. Oregon: Press Release; 2016. Available at: http://www.prweb.com/releases/2016/06/prweb13466816.htm.
4. Gulsvig J. Patient activation and engagement. Illinois: McKnight's; 2015. http://www.mcknights.com/marketplace/patient-activation-and-engagement/article/459663/.
5. Winner B, Peipert JF, Zhao Q, et al. Effectiveness of long-acting reversible contraception. N Engl J Med 2012;366(21):1998–2007.
6. Judith Hibbard, in an interview with the author, July 7, 2016.
7. Parekh AK. Winning their trust. N Engl J Med 2011;364(24):e51.
8. Shrank William H, Choudhry NK, Fischer MA, et al. The epidemiology of prescriptions abandoned at the pharmacy. Ann Intern Med 2010;153(10):633–40.

9. U.S. Department of Health and Human Services. Prevention makes common cents. Available at: https://aspe.hhs.gov/legacy-page/prevention-makes-common-cent-142526. Accessed June 14, 2016.

10. Hibbard JH, Greene J, Valerie O. Patients with lower activation associated with higher costs; delivery systems should know their patients' 'scores'. Health Aff 2013;32(2):216–22.

11. Hough DE. Irrationality in health care: what behavioral economics reveals about what we do and why. Stanford (CA): Stanford University Press; 2014.

12. Trzeciak S, Anthony M. Compassionomics: the revolutionary scientific evidence that caring makes a difference. Pensacola (FL): Studer Group Publishing; 2019.

13. Swayden KJ, Anderson KK, Connelly LM, et al. Effect of sitting vs. standing on perception of provider time at bedside: a pilot study. Patient Educ Couns 2012; 86(2):166–71.

14. Davis RE, Koutantji M, Vincent CA. How willing are patients to question healthcare staff on issues related to the quality and safety of their healthcare? An exploratory study. Qual Saf Health Care 2008;17(2):90–6.

15. Wolosin RJ, Vercler L, Matthews JL. "Am I safe here? Improving patients' perceptions of safety in hospitals. J Nurs Care Qual 2006;21(1):30–8 [quiz: 39–40].

Primary Care Transformation

Gregory Sawin, MD, MPH[a],*, Nicole O'Connor, MD[b]

KEYWORDS

- Primary care transformation • PCMH • Patient-centered • Team-based care

KEY POINTS

- In the United States, our hospital- and specialty-driven health system fueled by a fee-for-service model has created an expensive disease response system, but does not proactively promote health and wellness.
- Patient-centered care should be the guiding principle of transformation.
- Transformed primary care will have a laser-like focus on the patient experience of care and organize services to empower and engage patients to improve their health.
- Transformed care will get patients the right amount of care when and where it's needed.
- Patients need a system they trust to get the help they need in a timely manner. Transformed care will meet these needs and allow care to be escalated and deescalated seamlessly.

Primary care transformation, done right, will require a radical shift in the way we deliver health care in the United States. At more than $10,000 per capita, we spend the most on health care (over twice as much as an average wealthy nation),[1] and our performance is among the worst.[2] Many factors contribute to this dismal reality. At the foundation, the United States has built health care as a business, while public health is the domain of government.[3] The business has been built on a fee-for-service model that rewards clinicians when they do more (visits, tests, procedures) to patients, but does not actively promote health; it creates perverse disincentives, promotes waste, and discourages proactive prevention and population health management. In the crisis of our dysfunction that is fueling shifts to value-based care, we cannot afford not to increase investments in primary care. The value of excellent primary care is undeniable, and will play a central role in rescuing the failing US health care system.[4–8]

Disclosure Statement: The authors have nothing to disclose.
[a] Tufts University Family Medicine Residency, Malden Family Medicine Center, Cambridge Health Alliance, Tufts University School of Medicine, Harvard University Faculty of Medicine, 195 Canal Street, Malden, MA 02148, USA; [b] Practice Improvement Team, Patient Advisory Council, Tufts University Family Medicine Residency, Malden Family Medicine Center, Cambridge Health Alliance, Tufts University School of Medicine, 195 Canal Street, Malden, MA 02148, USA
* Corresponding author.
E-mail address: gsawin@challiance.org

Prim Care Clin Office Pract 46 (2019) 549–560
https://doi.org/10.1016/j.pop.2019.07.006
0095-4543/19/© 2019 Elsevier Inc. All rights reserved.

primarycare.theclinics.com

Primary care transformation needs to be driven by the guiding principles of patient centeredness and engagement. The challenge is to create a system that reliably and equitably provides the right amount of high quality care when and where it is needed. Meeting this challenge requires the building of authentic healing relationships, not just between patient and physician, but also between the patient and his or her health care team nested in a system that is robustly supported with sophisticated technology (**Box 1**).

To illustrate the radical patient centeredness required for primary care transformation, we have written 2 clinical vignettes (**Boxes 2** and **3**) to illustrate how transformed primary care will *feel* for our patients. Look for how these practices engage and empower patients and how connections and relationships are purposefully designed with health care team members and the technology to support it. Notice where the roles and systems reach for health beyond what we typically consider the purview of health care.

TEAM-BASED CARE

Most primary care offices practice in teams at some level; however, transformed primary care requires a new level of team performance. Practices will need to develop new roles and be integrated with other services and specialties including social services that will challenge our systems to reach for health beyond health care.[15] Teams will be oriented around a clear, shared vision of care that focuses on patient experience and engagement. The deep traditional hierarchies of medical care delivery will be challenged in high-functioning teams as broader arrays of staff are empowered to connect with patients.

Much has been written about various team configurations and roles in primary care, and those will certainly continue to evolve.[20] Specific needs of our patients (which will differ by community) should be the primary driver in the creation of new roles and services. Team member roles and duties should all be oriented around the concept of getting the right amount of care when and where it is needed, and distributing work such that all team members are spending most of their time working at the top of their skills and license capabilities.

One of the most promising developing roles in primary care is health coaching. Bellin Health has developed coaching within its care team coordinators (CTC) role. Bellin, and several other systems, have evolved these roles often by up-skilling medical assistants who are then deployed in a 2:1 ratio to providers.[9] CTCs do the typical medical assistant work of rooming and taking vitals, but also have expanded duties with agenda setting, addressing health maintenance, medication reconciliation, and support for health behavior change. When the clinician arrives, the CTC remains in the room, serves as scribe, and actively participates

---

Box 1
Key concepts for "transformed" primary care

1. Authentic healing relationships build trust.

2. Patients are confident their health care team will take excellent care of them.

3. The "system" delivers the right amount of care when and where it is needed.
   a. Patient-oriented technology (virtual visits and coaching)
   b. Escalation and deescalation as needed
   c. Broader roles and team members

Box 2
Chronic disease management

Mr. Rios: A 58 year-old man with diabetes, chronic obstructive pulmonary disease, hypertension, attempting smoking cessation.

Interviewer: Tell me about your last visit with your doctor.

Rios: I saw Dr. Klein 2 weeks ago, but Marina called me yesterday to see if I threw away all my ashtrays.

Interviewer: Who's Marina, and what's with the ashtrays?

Rios: She takes care of me. Dr. Klein calls her a care partner.[9] I call her my health coach![10,11]

A few years ago Dr. Klein's office started developing new roles. Marina was a medical assistant, but does a lot more now.

Interviewer: What changed?

Rios: One day she asked if it was okay if she stayed in the room to help with my appointment after she took my vitals. Marina helped me build a list of what I wanted to talk about, scheduled my colonoscopy, updated my medicines, and started talking about my smoking.

Interviewer: How was it with Marina in the visit?

Rios: I wasn't sure at first, but quickly realized it's a great thing. Dr. Klein listened better and wasn't so buried in the computer because Marina was taking the notes. When Dr. Klein was done, Marina had written everything down for me that I needed to remember and explained it all to me before I left—and then made me "teach back" to make sure I got it.[12] When Dr. Klein used to give me instructions at the end, she always seemed in a rush by the end of the visit. I know she's super busy, and I didn't want to slow her down, and also felt embarrassed if I didn't understand something.

Interviewer: What's the deal with the ashtray question?

Rios: I've been smoking for a long time and I know I need to quit, I really want to quit, but I wasn't sure if I'd be able to since I've been smoking so long. After my visit with Dr. Klein that day, Marina spent another 20 minutes with me developing a really detailed quit plan. How I'd take my medication, setting a quit date, making a big deal of it, telling my friends and family, and yes, throwing away my lighters and ashtrays to make a "nonsmoking house."[13] She told me she'd call me at 6 PM on my quit date, so I had an accountability piece built in to support me. She also got me set up with a smoking cessation group I'm meeting with weekly at the clinic. It's so great to go through this tough work with others wrestling with the same issue.[14] I've gone 46 days without a cigarette. I think I can do it for real this time!

Interviewer: How is your relationship with your primary care team now different than previous relationships you've had with a doctor?

Rios: I trust it. That's new for me. When I need something, I know I can call or send a message and Marina or whomever is covering for her will get back to me that day. They also lean into the hard stuff. Last year, they started using more questionnaires when I checked in. This one asked if I was having any trouble affording enough food, or medication or having trouble with my housing. I was too embarrassed to bring it up, but I was having trouble, and they introduced me to their Patient Resource Coordinator who got me set up with Meals on Wheels and sent a referral to the local food pantry.[15] They're not just pill pushers!

Interviewer: How do you contact them usually?

Rios: Marina helped me download an app to my phone. It was intimidating at first, but she showed me how to send questions, book appointments or refills. It's WAY more convenient than their old annoying phone tree.

Interviewer: But you still call them too.

Rios: Yeah, and their phone tree has gone away, so now when I call an actual person answers and tries to take care of everything I need on that same call so we're not playing an endless game of phone tag.

Interviewer: Are there others in the clinic you have relationships with?

Rios: Yes, Dr. Alex, she's a pharmacist who works with Dr. Klein. She taught me how to give myself insulin shots, which was scary at first. Since I have so much going on with my health, Alex has really focused on my diabetes and helped me get that much better under control.[16]

Interviewer: How was it different working with the pharmacist on your diabetes versus Dr. Klein?

Rios: We were focused on my diabetes. I always have 100 questions for Dr. Klein which quickly fills up my 20 minutes. My first visit with Dr. Alex was an hour and follow-up visits have been 30 minutes, I understand SO much more about my diabetes now.

Interviewer: It sounds like you really trust your primary care team. That's not always the case— how did they win your trust?

Rios: Same way we earn trust in any relationship, with time and reliability. I usually have trusted my doctor, but never their office staff.

Interviewer: What do you mean?

Rios: I've had some really good doctors, but like the annoying phone tree stuff, getting access to the doctor was a thrash and I didn't trust other folks in the office that they knew anything about me or my medical care. Now I'm okay talking with the person who answers the phone and telling her exactly what I need because she I know she'll make it happen, like make an appointment, get a refill, referral, whatever I need.

Interviewer: How does that feel having all these different folks take care of you?

Rios: I love it. Initially, I was suspicious of anyone besides Dr. Klein, but now I know I have a whole team that can take care of me and get me the right amount of care when and where I need it which is WAY more convenient than waiting for an appointment with my doctor for every little thing.

in the patient visit. Finally, when the provider finishes, the CTC reviews instructions, and arranges any follow-up or hand-offs. CTCs develop continuous relationships with the patients and serve as health coaches. Coaches provide self-management support, system navigation, emotional support, and help to bridge the gap between patient and clinician.[21] In a more traditional model, patients usually leave offices understanding only 50% of recommendations and instructions.[22] Coaching gives time and space for techniques like teach-back (ie, closed-loop communication) to increase patient understanding and empowerment.[12,23] These models increase provider and patient satisfaction, and improve performance metrics. Off-loaded tasks allow physicians on average to see one more patient per session, and the added revenue more than covers the cost of higher staffing ratios.[9,24]

As we develop a deeper focus on patient experience and engagement, we also need to think carefully about recruitment of our staff and leveraging their life experiences to build patient connection. Traditionally, we have focused on the doctor–patient relationship, which remains critical. Yet, as we think about partnering more comprehensively with patients, we must rely more on our team members. Community health worker models are some of the most advanced in this arena of purposeful recruiting, training, and ongoing support. They underscore that the best individuals to connect with patients in the community are folks from the community who have a shared life experience. Shifting the focus to hiring for the *who* and training and

Box 3
Expanding concepts of access and visits: the right amount of care when and where it's needed

Ms. Corbett: A 32-year-old mother of 3- and 6-year-old children who are also patients in the practice.

Interviewer. Tell me about your last interaction with your primary care doctor.

Corbett: Last week, I sent a message to the office on MyChart because I noticed burning when I urinated and I was going more than usual.

Interviewer. What is MyChart?

Corbett: It's a website and app I can use to send messages to the office and see a lot of info about my health care.

Interviewer: What happened after you sent the message?

Corbett: Christine, the nurse on my team, called me with a few more questions about my symptoms. She thought I had a urinary tract infection and sent in a prescription for an antibiotic.

Interviewer: Did you talk to Dr. Early?

Corbett: No, only Christine.

Interviewer: How do you feel about not talking to your doctor directly when you're not feeling well?

Corbett: Great. I know Christine. She did my first prenatal visits and has worked there for a long time. She answers my MyChart messages for me and my kids and I know she works very closely with Dr. Early, who could be hard to reach, so I get what I need more quickly instead of waiting for a day or two for Dr. Early to get back to me. It takes a lot of time, effort, and money to get into the clinic with 2 young kids or to get a babysitter, so when I can get care I trust without coming in, that's great!

Interviewer: Are there times when you've sent a message and the team asked you to come in?

Corbett: Yes, after my second baby I got depressed. I sent a message to Dr. Early saying I was feeling sad and having trouble caring for my son. Christine got the message and called me right away. She asked me a bunch of questions to make sure I was safe and then scheduled an appointment the next morning with Dr. Early.

Interviewer: Wow, you were able to get care very quickly.

Corbett: Yes, I was surprised by how quickly Christine called and was able to get an appointment. She said it was urgent, and keeps a few appointments open for these types of things.[16] Also, if I didn't have this depth of relationship with my health care team, I don't think I would have felt comfortable telling them how bad I was feeling, but I knew they cared and would want to know.

Interviewer: So you have meaningful relationships with more team members than just your primary care doctor? Tell me more about that.

Corbett: Besides Christine, I know the medical assistant, Toni, who works with Dr. Early. I see her every time the kids or I have appointments. She gets us settled, makes sure we're updated on our vaccines and check-ups. She sent a message last week reminding me to schedule my daughter's physical, and asked how I was doing after I took the antibiotics for the urinary tract infection.

Interviewer: How is your relationship with this team different from previous relationships you've had with a doctor or health system?

Corbett: My doctor works with a team of people who seem to really know me and my family. I usually see or speak with the same few people; they know my story, or at least have easy access to my record, and seem to know me, so I don't have to start from scratch with every conversation. They're seamless, I get answers when I call or send a message and don't feel lost like I did with other health systems. I'm a lot less frantic about getting care. In the past I didn't have confidence that my doctor and the health system would proactively take care of me, so I had to be a really staunch self-advocate. Which sometimes made me get more care than I actually needed. In the past, I was always ending up in the emergency room with my oldest who has asthma. That doesn't happen anymore. She has a care plan we all understand. I trust my team. If something can be handled without a visit, that's better for all of us, and if I need more help, I know I'll get that too.

Interviewer: It sounds like you really trust your primary care team, that's not always the case. How did they win your trust?

Corbett: I felt like the team really cared when I sent the message that I was feeling sad after my son was born. Christine called me to check in and get me an appointment right away. Dr. Early knew why I was coming in and asked a psychologist, Dr. Zona, to come and speak with me while I was there.[17] I was really nervous about seeing a psychologist. But having Dr. Early introduce her and being able to see her at my regular clinic made it a lot easier. I saw Dr. Zona for a couple months and felt a lot better. I haven't felt taken care of like that by anyone in health care before.

Interviewer: What happens when you need care that is, beyond what Dr. Early can provide?

Corbett: Dr. Early or the team can order the usual referrals, like seeing the psychologist, but she's also been able to get help without seeing a specialist. When I was depressed, we tried a couple different medications but I had a lot of side effects from them and was nervous about trying new medications because I was breastfeeding. It was a really long wait to see a psychiatrist to help figure out medication. So Dr. Early made an e-consult with a psychiatrist who recommended a medication change after reviewing my chart.[18,19] I didn't have to wait months and it saved me a visit and co-pay.

Interviewer: Are there other instances where you've been able to get specialty help like that?

Corbett: Yes, a few months ago my daughter had a rash on her arm that wouldn't go away. We were traveling and I wasn't able to bring her in, so I sent a photo through MyChart to Dr. Early to see if she could tell us what to do. She sent it to the dermatologist to review and sent me back recommendations. It was so easy and we were able to enjoy our trip.

Interviewer: Sounds like you love MyChart. Is this the main way you communicate with the office?

Corbett: Yes, the patient portal system is super easy to use, so I prefer that over the phone. I can log in on my computer or use the app on my phone and send messages after hours, as long as they're not emergencies. Then I don't have to worry about going back and forth leaving messages or only being able to ask a question before 5 PM The messages seem to get to the right person reliably. I can also look at notes from our visits or the kids' vaccination records.

supporting for the *what* of the work bolsters the roles to create higher functioning teams.[25] This is also a crucial strategy to increase health equity and decrease disparities.

AUTHENTIC HEALING RELATIONSHIPS

Authentic healing relationships are characterized by the core elements of security, genuineness, and continuity.[17] They work by "(1) valuing/creating a nonjudgmental emotional bond; (2) appreciating power/consciously managing clinician power in ways that would most benefit the patient; and (3) abiding/displaying a commitment to caring for patients over time."[16] Traditionally, we have thought about these relationships as existing only between a healer and patient, but with new team-based models, these relationships will also need to develop between the team and patient. Patients may have greater rapport with their health coach than they do with their clinician. This relationship shift may feel like a loss to physicians in transformed primary care. The traditional physician-centric model where doctors are the virtuoso violin player must evolve so they are effective team leaders working instead as orchestra conductors. With an estimated shortage of primary care physicians reaching 44,000 by 2035, models must leverage other roles to build the meaningful relationships patients need.[26]

TECHNOLOGY

Transformed primary care will harness the power of technology to nurture relationships. As illustrated in the vignette in **Box 2**, technology can allow systems to improve access, right-size care, and share information among teams and patients. Patient-facing technology includes patient portals, information-gathering devices, and personalized coaching and advice. Patient portals enable asynchronous visits with care teams that can improve patient satisfaction and increase the efficiency and quality of face-to-face visits.[27] Data sharing, including patient input of blood pressure, blood sugar, weight, and other information can improve self-management of chronic disease.[28] As patient portals become more sophisticated, abnormal values can trigger urgent responses from team members as well as access to curated health education. Similarly, as smart devices, such as phones, activity trackers, and watches evolve, greater automation of data collection and sharing will enable teams to provide customized care. Bidirectional data sharing through shared record keeping such as

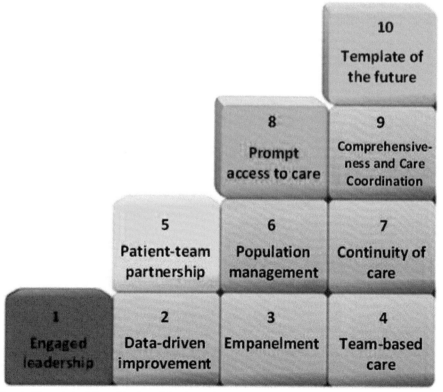

Fig. 1. The 10 building blocks of high-performing primary care. ©2012 UCSF Center for Excellence in Primary Care.

open notes provides transparency for patients to review their visits, keep goals aligned, and empower patients to help direct their own care.[29]

Electronic medical records (EMRs) support population health management by generating registries for chronic diseases and preventive care. As EMRs advance, actionable reports will allow team members to proactively address population health as they communicate with each other around outreach, and progress toward goals, which can increase engagement and improve outcomes in chronic disease management.[29] On a broader level, metadata from EMRs can help to identify disease trends and resource needs to direct health care and public health systems to better serve patients and communities.[30]

TRANSFORMATION MODELS

Each practice, health system and community will have unique characteristics that must be considered as they transform their care models. Thankfully, primary care transformation has been well studied, and there are excellent models that can provide a road map and tools to help practices evolve. Two leading models are *The 10 Building Blocks of High-Performing Primary Care* from the University of California–San Francisco Center for Excellence in Primary Care[31] and the Qualis Health's *Safety Net Medical Home Initiative*,[32] which similarly organizes steps of transformation into *Change Concepts* that are sequenced in a particular order to increase chances of success.

There are many commonalities between the 2 models, including the need for engaged leadership, adoption of a shared model for data-driven improvement,

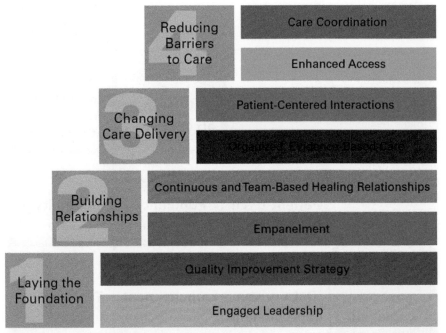

Fig. 2. Safety net medical home initiative: change concepts. (*From* Sugarman JR, Phillips KE, Wagner EH, et al. The Safety Net Medical Home Initiative: transforming care for vulnerable populations. Med Care. 2014;52:S3; with permission.)

empanelment, team-based care, panel management, and advanced access. Each of these models has a collection of interactive tools and materials that can provide structure and support for practices ready to engage in an active transformation efforts (**Figs. 1** and **2**).[33,34]

Practice transformation must be seen as a long journey; many "transformed practices" unfold over a 3- to 5-year period. Indeed, a culture of continual improvement will keep practices evolving to better meet patient needs.[35] Most health care professionals have not received training in improvement science, which is a critical skill needed to support transformation. Whether health care professionals adopt the models mentioned, or Lean or Six Sigma,[36] or another model entirely, the "secret sauce" that makes any model work includes 3 key ingredients: (1) the discipline of building a shared language and improvement practices, (2) being data driven, and (3) empowering everyone on the team to pose the orienting question of the Institute for Healthcare Improvement's Model for Improvement[37]: "What are we trying to accomplish?" Similarly, team members should all make contributions unique to each person's perspective.[37] Practice transformation collaboratives can be effective strategies to grow improvement capacity and to provide technical assistance and coaching for clinics to evolve.[38,39]

SUMMARY

Primary care transformation should be driven by the guiding principle that all people deserve an authentic healing relationship with a primary care team they trust will take excellent care of them. The primary care team is the patient's first point of contact with the health system supported by relationships that are long term and provide continuity, and a proactive person (not disease) focus of care.[40] These concepts are not new in primary care, but also have not been supported to grow to fruition as the underfunded "step-child" of a fee-for-service health system.

Our practices need to lean in to intentionally build relationships so our patients feel known, understood, and trust that we will take care of them. Getting the right amount of care when and where it is needed empowers patients to navigate their needs. Tools can help; robust patient portals, convenient apps that promote engagement, activity trackers, and smart devices that push information into our EMRs and nudge them to make healthier decisions all have promise. Behind the scenes, health systems must be able to accurately assess patient needs, linking them efficiently to appropriate services, whether gentle reassurance for a cold, an e-consult with a specialist, a visit with their primary care provider, advice for an emergency room visit, or a referral to a local food pantry. In our current catastrophic care model, many of these simple concerns wind up in wasteful emergency room visits. As illustrated in the vignettes, relationships are changing to leverage other caregivers beyond the primary care physician, and technology will also play a key role in facilitating those interactions. If we ask, patients will guide our way and should be aggressively recruited to participate in our planning and design with attention to the concept of co-production of health.[41–43]

ACKNOWLEDGMENTS

Thomas Bodenheimer, MD, is Founding Director, Center for Excellence in Primary Care, University of California, San Francisco. Allen Shaughnessy, PharmD, MMedEd, is Director, Master Teacher Fellowship, Professor and Vice Chair of Family Medicine for Research Tufts University School of Medicine.

REFERENCES

1. Papanicolas I, Woskie LR, Jha AK. Health care spending in the united states and other high-income countries. JAMA 2018;319(10):1024–39.
2. Anderson G, Hussey PS. Comparing health system performance in OECD countries. Health Aff (Millwood) 2001;20(3):219–32.
3. Landon BE, Grumbach K, Wallace PJ. Integrating public health and primary care systems: potential strategies from an IOM report. JAMA 2012;308(5):461–2.
4. Bindman AB, Grumbach K, Osmond D, et al. Primary care and receipt of preventive services. J Gen Intern Med 1996;11(5):269–76.
5. Safran DG, Taira DA, Rogers WH, et al. Linking primary care performance to outcomes of care. J Fam Pract 1998;47(3):213.
6. Stewart AL, Grumbach K, Osmond DH, et al. Primary care and patient perceptions of access to care. J Fam Pract 1997;44(2):177.
7. Rosenblatt RA, Hart LG, Baldwin L-M, et al. The generalist role of specialty physicians: is there a hidden system of primary care? JAMA 1998;279(17):1364–70.
8. Macinko J, Starfield B, Shi L. The contribution of primary care systems to health outcomes within organization for economic cooperation and development (OECD) countries, 1970–1998. Health Serv Res 2003;38(3):831–65.
9. Bodenheimer T, Syer S. Bright spo... tinsprimary care: 7.
10. Gastala N, Wingrove P, Gaglioti A, et al. The growing trend of health coaches in team-based primary care training a multicenter pilot study. Fam Med 2018. https://doi.org/10.22454/FamMed.2018.459897.
11. Ghorob A. SUPPLEMENT: health coaching: teaching patients to fish. Fam Pract Manag 2013;20(3):40–2.
12. Bodenheimer T. Teach-back: a simple technique to enhance patients' understanding. Fam Pract Manag 2018;25(4):20–2.
13. Interprofessional collaboration regarding patients' care plans in primary care: a focus group study into influential factors | BMC Family Practice | Full Text. Available at: https://bmcfampract-biomedcentral-com.ezproxy.library.tufts.edu/articles/10.1186/s12875-016-0456-5. Accessed February 7, 2019.
14. Kirsh SR, Aron DC, Johnson KD, et al. A realist review of shared medical appointments: how, for whom, and under what circumstances do they work? BMC Health Serv Res 2017;17(1):113.
15. DeVoe JE, Bazemore AW, Cottrell EK, et al. Perspectives in primary care: a conceptual framework and path for integrating social determinants of health into primary care practice. Ann Fam Med 2016;14(2):104–8.
16. Ansell D, Crispo JAG, Simard B, et al. Interventions to reduce wait times for primary care appointments: a systematic review. BMC Health Serv Res 2017;17(1):295.
17. Cohen DJ, Balasubramanian BA, Davis M, et al. Understanding care integration from the ground up: five organizing constructs that shape integrated practices. J Am Board Fam Med 2015;28(Supplement 1):S7–20.
18. Electronic consultation systems: worldwide prevalence and their impact on patient care—a systematic review | Family Practice | Oxford Academic. Available at: https://academic-oup-com.ezproxy.library.tufts.edu/fampra/article/33/3/274/1749814. Accessed February 7, 2019.
19. Rodriguez KL, Burkitt KH, Bayliss NK, et al. Veteran, primary care provider, and specialist satisfaction with electronic consultation. JMIR Med Inform 2015;3(1). https://doi.org/10.2196/medinform.3725.

20. Wagner EH, Flinter M, Hsu C, et al. Effective team-based primary care: observations from innovative practices. BMC Fam Pract 2017;18(1). https://doi.org/10.1186/s12875-017-0590-8.
21. Bennett HD, Coleman EA, Parry C, et al. Health coaching for patients with chronic illness. Fam Pract Manag 2010;17(5):24.
22. Bodenheimer T. A 63-year-old man with multiple cardiovascular risk factors and poor adherence to treatment Plans. JAMA 2007;298(17):2048–55.
23. Badaczewski A, Bauman LJ, Blank AE, et al. Relationship between Teach-back and patient-centered communication in primary care pediatric encounters. Patient Educ Couns 2017;100(7):1345–52.
24. Lyon C, English AF, Smith PC. A team-based care model that improves Job satisfaction. Fam Pract Manag 2018;25(2):6–11.
25. Community Health Worker Toolkit. Available at: http://www.health.state.mn.us/divs/orhpc/workforce/emerging/chw/2016chwtool.pdf. Accessed January 30, 2019.
26. Petterson SM, Liaw WR, Tran C, et al. Estimating the residency expansion required to avoid projected primary care physician shortages by 2035. Ann Fam Med 2015;13(2):107–14.
27. Wade-Vuturo AE, Mayberry LS, Osborn CY. Secure messaging and diabetes management: experiences and perspectives of patient portal users. J Am Med Inform Assoc 2013;20(3):519–25.
28. Urowitz S, Wiljer D, Dupak K, et al. Improving diabetes management with a patient portal: qualitative study of a diabetes self-management portal. J Med Internet Res 2012;14(6). https://doi.org/10.2196/jmir.2265.
29. Ngui D, Qiu MJH, Mann M. OS 26-04 targeting care gaps in patients with hypertension: a quality improvement project utilizing EMR hypertension dashboards and a chronic disease coordinator. J Hypertens 2016;34:e247.
30. Bazemore AW, Cottrell EK, Gold R, et al. "Community vital signs": incorporating geocoded social determinants into electronic records to promote patient and population health. J Am Med Inform Assoc 2016;23(2):407–12.
31. Bodenheimer T, Ghorob A, Willard-Grace R, et al. The 10 building blocks of high-performing primary care. Ann Fam Med 2014;12(2):166–71.
32. Sugarman JR, Phillips KE, Wagner EH, et al. The safety net medical home initiative: transforming care for vulnerable populations. Med Care 2014;52:S1–10.
33. Tools for Transformation | Center for Excellence in Primary Care. Available at: https://cepc.ucsf.edu/tools-transformation. Accessed January 29, 2019.
34. Resources & Tools | Safety Net Medical Home Initiative. Available at: http://www.safetynetmedicalhome.org/resources-tools. Accessed January 29, 2019.
35. Crabtree BF, Nutting PA, Miller WL, et al. Summary of the national demonstration project and recommendations for the patient-centered medical home. Ann Fam Med 2010;8(Suppl 1):S80–90.
36. What is Lean Healthcare? NEJM Catalyst. 2018. Available at: https://catalyst.nejm.org/what-is-lean-healthcare/. Accessed February 8, 2019.
37. Institute for Healthcare Improvement. How to improve. Available at: http://www.ihi.org:80/resources/Pages/HowtoImprove/default.aspx. Accessed February 7, 2019.
38. Grumbach K, Mold JW. A health care cooperative extension service: transforming primary care and community health. JAMA 2009;301(24):2589–91.
39. Bitton A, Ellner A, Pabo E, et al. The Harvard Medical School academic innovations collaborative: transforming primary care practice and education. Acad Med 2014;89(9):1239.

40. Medicine I of. Primary care: America's health in a new era 2001. https://doi.org/10.17226/5152.
41. DiGioia AM, Shapiro E. The patient centered value system. New York: transforming healthcare through Co-design. Taylor & Francis; 2017. Available at: https://books.google.com/books?id=E3BQDwAAQBAJ.
42. Nelson EC, Batalden PB, Godfrey MM, et al. Value by design: developing clinical microsystems to achieve organizational excellence. Wiley; 2011. Available at: https://books.google.com/books?id=I3GhR3-IgTgC.
43. Batalden P. Getting more health from healthcare: quality improvement must acknowledge patient coproduction—an essay by Paul Batalden. BMJ 2018; 362:k3617.

Assessing and Addressing Social Determinants of Health

A Key Competency for Succeeding in Value-Based Care

Jennifer Houlihan, MSP[a],*, Steve Leffler, MD[b]

KEYWORDS

- Social determinants of health • Innovation • Return on investment

KEY POINTS

- Social determinants represent 40% to 50% of the cost structure in Medicare and Medicaid.
- Incorporating social determinants of health (SDH) into strategy and care model design is emerging as a key factor in identifying and managing patient risk.
- Health systems are investing in several innovative social determinant initiatives; major themes include a focus on addressing food security and housing.
- Scalability remains a challenge given where providers and health systems are in the transition to value; estimating cost avoidance/savings to a health system is key in generating support for models.
- Predictive models and CMS-endorsed screening tools are beginning to influence a more standardized approach to screening for SDH in the electronic health record (EHR) as part of the patient visit.

INTRODUCTION

According to a 2018 Physicians Foundation *Survey of America's Physicians*, nearly 90% of US physicians report that some of their patients have a social condition that affects their health, whether it be unemployment, lack of education, or drug addiction.[1] With the transition toward value-based payments, the need to focus efforts on reducing health spending by improving health outcomes highlights the need for

Disclosure: The authors have nothing to disclose.
[a] Wake Forest Baptist Medical Center, CIN-Population Health, Medical Center Boulevard, Winston-Salem, NC 27157, USA; [b] University of Vermont Health Network, The University of Vermont Medical Center, 111 Colchester Avenue – 101PA3, Burlington, VT 05401, USA
* Corresponding author.
E-mail address: jhouliha@wakehealth.edu

physicians and care teams to pay more attention to the social, economic, and environmental factors influencing their patients' health.

The World Health Organization defines social determinants of health (SDH) as the conditions in which people are born, grow, live, work, and age.

- Economic stability (poverty, employment, food security, and housing stability)
- Education (high school graduation, enrollment in higher education, and language and literacy)
- Social and community context (social cohesion, discrimination, and incarceration)
- Health and health care (accessibility and health literacy)
- Neighborhood and built environment (food deserts, quality of housing, and safety)
- It is anticipated that the sixth SDH factor is access to broadband. The American Medical Informatics Association has stated that it "believe[s] that access to broadband is, or will soon become, a social determinant of health." Lacking access to reliable and affordable Internet or mobile service limits not only a person's ability to use technology for health-related purposes but also their ability to access other important services, such as emergency assistance or employment opportunities.

SDH are the factors mostly responsible for health inequities—the avoidable differences in health status seen within and between different geographic locations.[2] The Healthy People 2020 initiative defines 5 broad SDH factors as depicted in **Fig. 1.**[3]

The United States is the highest health spender among Organization for Economic Co-operation and Development (OECD) countries at $9086 per person and yet has worse population health outcomes when compared with its international counterparts. The OECD has reported that the United States spends the largest share of its gross domestic product on health care, at 17%, and is ranked 23rd of 34 nations in terms of social service spending.[4] In the United States, place of birth is more strongly associated with life expectancy than race or genetics.[3] On average, there is a 15-year difference in life expectancy between the most advantaged and disadvantaged citizens.[4] This difference is correlated with geographic characteristics and health behaviors[5]

Economic Stability	Education	Community & Social Context	Health Care System	Neighborhood & Built Environment
• Employment • Income • Medical Debt • Expenses	• Literacy • Language • Higher Education • Early Childhood Education • Vocational Training	• Social Integration • Community Engagement • Support Systems • Discrimination	• Healthcare Coverage • Provider Availability • Provider Cultural Competency • Quality of Care	• Housing • Transportation • Food/Access to Healthy Options • Safety • Parks/ Playgrounds • Walkability
Health Outcomes				
Mortality Life Expectancy Healthcare Expenditures Health Status Functional Limitations				

Fig. 1. Social determinants of health. (*Adapted from* Artiga S, Hinton E. Beyond healthcare: the role of social determinants in promoting health and health equity. Available at: https://www.kff.org/disparities-policy/issue-brief/beyond-health-care-the-role-of-social-determinants-in-promoting-health-and-health-equity/; with permission.)

that are influenced by historical and social factors. Population-level inequalities in health care result in $309 billion in losses to the economy annually, and disproportionately affect disadvantaged populations.[6] Research shows that health care is just one of many health determinants, because it is suggested that greater than 80% of patient health is determined by the SDH (**Fig. 2**) as opposed to genetic makeup or other health-related factors such as health care access.[6]

For the first time in our history, the United States is raising a generation of children who may live sicker and shorter lives than their parents. Reversing this trend will of course depend on healthy choices by each of us. But not everyone in America has the same opportunities to be healthy.

According to the most recent data available from the Centers for Disease Control and Prevention, average life expectancy in the United States is 78.6 years— 76.1 years for men and 81.1 years for women, down 0.3 years from 2015.[7] Adding to a 2017 analysis that found growing disparities in life expectancy across US counties and zip codes, the National Center for Health Statistics has released first-of-its-kind neighborhood-level data on life expectancy at birth, which shows that life expectancy estimates vary greatly even at the census tract level, from block to block. Developed with support from the Robert Wood Johnson Foundation, the data make it possible to understand how much our health is influenced by the conditions we experience where we live.

For the first time in history, in the United States life expectancy for children is now shorter than their patients, an indication of the nation's overall health.

In recognition of the strong link between SDH and health care, the Health Resources & Services Administration's Office of Health Equity has recognized SDH as vital to population health. With social determinants representing 40% to 50% of the cost structure in Medicare and Medicaid, CMS (Center for Medicaid and Medicare Services) has also recognized that managing SDH is key to controlling the cost of health care.[8] In 2010, Congress passed the Patient Protection and Affordable Care Act to

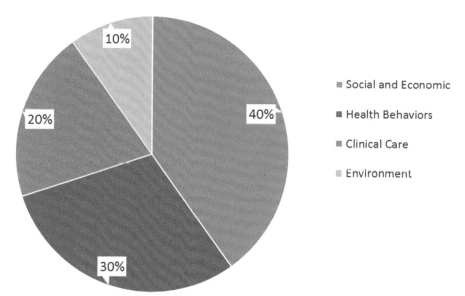

Fig. 2. Factors affecting health. (*Data from* Hood CM, Gennuso KP, Swain GR, et al. County health rankings: relationships between determinant factors and health outcomes. Am J Prev Med. 2016;50(2):129-35.)

promote overall public health, recognizing the health disparities associated with people not having health coverage because of low incomes and/or preexisting medical conditions. The law established a $10 billion Prevention and Public Health Fund to expand national investments in prevention and public health and improve health outcomes.

PAYER AND PROVIDER TRANSFORMATION IN SOCIAL DETERMINANTS OF HEALTH

With health leaders recognizing that value-based care and controlling the cost of care cannot be achieved without addressing SDH, payers, providers, and government entities are investing in new innovations and strategic partnerships to advance health care beyond the traditional clinic and hospital setting. An outline of key emerging trends advancing the integration of SDH over the next decade are outlined in **Table 1**.

Social Determinants of Health Informing Patient Risk

Under risk adjustment, an Accountable Care Organization (ACO) or insurer who enrolls a greater than average number of high-risk individuals receives compensation to make up for extra costs associated with those enrollees. These models often account for patients' medical histories and factor in chronic conditions. By incorporating social determinants into risk-adjustment formulas, the accuracy of the relative rates could be increased. Beginning in 2019, the CMS will incorporate socioeconomic status of dual-eligible (beneficiaries are eligible for Medicare and Medicaid) patients toward

Table 1	
Emerging social determinants of health trends in payer and provider transformation	
Using SDH to inform patient risk	Risk-adjustment models that incorporate SDH can improve accuracy related to payment, and patients identified for care management interventions.
Health plan benefits address social determinants	Medicare Advantage plans have greater flexibility in offering benefits that address SDH.
Investing and partnering with community organizations	Payers are increasing investments in community agencies that address SDH, such as food insecurity and homelessness/housing.
States requiring SDH screening as part of Medicaid	Approximately 40% of US States now require that Medicaid Managed Care plans screen for SDH.
Availability/type of SDH screening tools consolidating and advanced analytical capabilities	SDH screening tools are becoming more nationally aligned with CMS guidelines adopted in EMRs along with predictive analytics, network registries of community-based organizations, and referral platforms as part of care management solutions.
CMS innovation models and funding targeted toward addressing SDH	The Accountable Communities for Health Model is testing SDH screening with 31 organizations nationally.
Provider-led care management team and workflows updated to incorporate SDH	Updated care team models use SDH data to direct the work of social workers, health coaches, nutritionists, and pharmacists to work within and outside the health system to coordinate and manage care.

readmissions.[9] Dual-eligibles' tend to have fragmented care, leading to higher use of health services and is considered a proxy for socioeconomic status. The incorporation of SDH in patient risk may allow for more accurate payment amounts and could also inform patient panel size and compensation models under future value-based payment models.

Health Plan Benefits Address Social Determinants

In April 2018, CMS issued a final rule giving Medicare Advantage plans additional flexibility in determining supplemental benefits to include items and services to address SDH. CMS is beginning to address the existing standards for supplemental benefits to include additional services that "increase health and improve quality of life, including coverage of non-skilled in-home supports and other assistive devices."[10] Changes to the Medicare Advantage program present opportunities for plans to address some social needs, including offering supplemental benefits that support Activities of Daily Living and Instrumental Activities of Daily Living (eg, transportation to health care appointments, home safety modifications).

Investing and Partnering with Community Organizations

According to *8th Annual Industry Pulse Report*, payers are taking action to address SDH through community programs and screenings as a way to support value-based care initiatives. Forty-two percent of payers surveyed are integrating community programs and resources into their population health strategies including funding.[11] For example, the Humana Foundation has invested nearly $7 million in 9 organizations that are committed to addressing SDH, including food security, social connection, and financial stability. The investments include a donation to the San Antonio Food Bank to help create a Senior Wellness Intervention Model program to reduce food insecurity and social isolation. Investments in San Antonio's Older Adults Technology Services were also made to help alleviate social isolation among seniors through free access to Internet-connected technology. Other examples include Kaiser Permanente announcing a $200 million investment to combat homelessness, and the Blue Cross Blue Shield of North Carolina announcing an investment of $50 million in community health initiatives focused on 4 areas: addressing the state's opioid epidemic, early childhood development, SDH, and primary care.

State Medicaid Requirements Require Social Determinants of Health Screening

State Medicaid agencies are increasingly mandating that SDH be addressed in an effort to provide more efficient care and improve health outcomes. CMS regulations in May 2016 modernized Medicaid Managed Care operations (MCOs), accountability, and oversight.[12] **Box 1** provides more detail regarding the Medicaid SDH requirements in 5 States. One aspect of the modernization included promoting practices to address the social and structural factors of poverty, access to stable housing, social support networks, exposure to environmental toxins or community violence, and systematic discrimination. In 2018, approximately 40% of US States required MCOs to screen beneficiaries for social needs and/or provide enrollees with referrals to social services.[13]

The 2017, the Kaiser Family Foundation conducted a survey of 280 Medicaid Managed Care plans, with survey results indicating that screening and linking to social services were the predominant strategies with almost all plans (91%) reporting activities to address SDH, with housing, nutrition/food security, and education reported as top targets, as depicted in **Fig. 3**.

Box 1
Examples of States integrating social determinants into Medicaid Managed Care contracts

- Arizona requires coordination of community resources, such as housing and utility assistance, under its managed long-term services and supports contract. The state provides state-only funding in conjunction with its managed behavioral health contract to provide housing assistance.

- The District of Columbia encourages MCOs to refer beneficiaries with 3 or more chronic conditions to the "My Health GPS" Health Home program for care coordination and case-management services, including a biopsychosocial needs assessment and referral to community and social support services.

- Louisiana requires its plans to screen for problem gaming and tobacco use, and requires referrals to the Special Supplemental Nutrition Program for Women, Infants, and Children and the Louisiana Permanent Supportive Housing program when appropriate.

- Nebraska requires MCOs to have staff trained on SDH and be familiar with community resources; plans are also required to have policies to address members with multiple biopsychosocial needs.

- North Carolina requires participating MCOs to use a standardized statewide screening tool covering housing, food, transportation, and interpersonal violence to identify patients' unmet health-related resource needs. Patients will then be connected to appropriate community resources through a statewide platform being funded and developed by a public-private partnership.

Kaiser Family Foundation managed care initiatives; and *Data from* Crumley D, Lloyd J, Pucciarello M, et al. Addressing social determinants of health via Medicaid managed care contracts and Section 115 demonstrations. Available at: https://www.chcs.org/resource/addressing-social-determinants-of-health-via-medicaid-managed-care-contracts-and-section-1115-demonstrations/.

Social Determinants of Health Screening Tools and Advanced Analytics

Emerging technology solutions include predictive analytics, network registries of community-based organizations, and referral platforms as part of care management solutions. The engagement of advanced analytics to identify risk factors and provide prescriptive analytics to proactively address gaps in care can contribute to

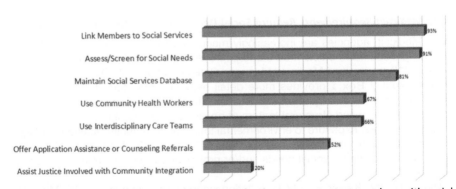

Fig. 3. Strategies Medicaid Managed Care Organization use to connect members with social services. (*Data from* Garfield R, Hinton E, Cornachione E, et al. Medicaid managed care plans and access to care. Available at: http://files.kff.org/attachment/Report-Medicaid-Managed-Care-March-Plans-and-Access-to-Care.)

decrease treatment costs by proactively identifying and handling health issues before they become a serious health crisis including reducing hospital readmissions.

In 2013, the National Association of Community Health Centers, the Association of Asian Pacific Community Health Organizations, the Oregon Primary Care Association, and the Institute for Alternative Futures collaborated to develop a standardized assessment tool known as the Protocol for Responding to and Assessing Patients' Assets, Risks, and Experiences.[14] Health Leads, a national health care organization that connects low-income patients with the basic resources they need to be healthy, created a screening toolkit that guides providers in how to ask questions to uncover underlying social needs, and gauges the impact of these needs on health and well-being. More recently, the Center for Medicare and Medicaid Innovation released an Accountable Health Communities screening tool that was tested by a panel of experts to identify patients' unmet needs. SDH screening tools are increasingly being incorporated into payer and health system initiatives to proactively identify patients by level of social risk. Despite the importance of SDH data, and recent policy emphasis on health care providers collecting and acting on SDH, the process has been gradual with no one standardized approach, and will likely evolve as integration continues to occur. A comparison of the key domains screened for in SDH automated/EMR tools is provided in **Table 2**.[15]

Center for Medicaid and Medicare Services Innovation Models

The CMS AHC Model is testing whether universal screening for health-related social needs and enhanced clinical-community linkages can improve health outcomes and reduce costs for Medicare and commercially insured beneficiaries. Nationwide, 31 organizations are providing support to community bridge organizations to test promising service delivery approaches aimed at linking beneficiaries with community services that may address their health-related social needs (ie, housing instability, food insecurity, utility needs, interpersonal violence, and transportation needs).[16]

Provider-Led Care Management Team and Workflows

Increasing payer and governmental focus on SDH will place more responsibilities on physicians as they manage care teams that become responsible for administering screening assessments and referring patients to community resources for identified issues. Providers administering SDH assessments will need to establish new workflows to track patient needs and referrals. These efforts will help to standardize the process of screening patients and referring to services along with using a comprehensive care team model to better understand team members' roles and responsibilities.[15] Updated care team models include the use of social workers, health coaches, nutritionists, and pharmacists to work within and outside the health system to coordinate and manage care. Establishing a consistent approach to measurement ensures that patients are assessed at appropriate intervals to track changes in health condition, social needs, goals, and referrals.

PROMISING PRACTICES: PROVIDER HEALTH SYSTEM SOCIAL DETERMINANTS OF HEALTH MODELS

A 2017 survey of 300 hospitals and health systems by The Deloitte Center for Health Solutions study on SDH found that the vast majority were committed to addressing social determinants and were screening patients for social needs.

Table 2
SDH tool comparison example

Domain	CMS AHC Screening Tool	PRAPARE Tool	Health Leads Social Assessment
Alcohol/Substance Use	X		Optional
Race/Ethnicity		X	X
Geography/Zip Code		X	X
Housing Instability	X	X	X
Income		X	X
Employment	X	X	Optional
Mental Health/ Depression	X		Optional
Education	X	X	
Financial Resource Strain	X	X	X
Food Insecurity	X	X	X
Intimate Partner Violence	X	X	X
Physical Activity	X		Optional
Family or Social Support	X	X	Optional
Stress		X	X
Transportation	X	X	X
Other	Disabilities; Utilities	Language preference, Veteran status, Refugee, Seasonal or farmworker status as main source of income; Incarceration history	Utilities

Abbreviations: AHC, Accountable Health Communities; PRAPARE, protocol for responding to and assessing patients' assets, risks, and experiences.

Adapted from Thomas-Henkel C, Schulman M. Screening for social determinants of health in populations with complex needs: implementation considerations. Available at: https://www.chcs.org/media/SDOH-Complex-Care-Screening-Brief-102617.pdf; with permission.

However, sustainable funding remained a challenge. As a result, most systems have limited their activities to target a small subset of their patient populations, such as high users, or those who are at risk of becoming frequent emergency department visitors.[17] With many systems transitioning to value-based care, innovations and investments in SDH are increasingly viewed as essential to a comprehensive population health strategy. As hospitals and health systems bear more risk and/or develop their own insurance plans, the incentive to provide care in the most cost-effective and potent manner will only continue to underscore the importance of social determinants. Several examples of innovative health system programming that address SDH include the following:

- Advocate Health Care, Illinois: implements quality improvement initiatives within their ACO to target malnutrition and food insufficiency. The ACO completed a screening of all patients at risk for malnutrition, with individuals with elevated risk scores receiving an oral nutritional supplement within 2 days of admission. Within the first 6 months, the ACO reduced health care costs by $3800 per patient, resulting in $4.8 million in total savings.[18]

- Atrium Health, North Carolina: collects demographic data from various sources including local universities and public health departments with a goal of identifying, cataloging, and documenting patient social determinant information to then connect them with community supports. Atrium's food insecurity screening pilot project targets senior patients at highest risk for readmissions and provides emergency food services and helps them complete the Supplemental Nutrition Assistance Program applications. As a result, Atrium Health has reduced readmissions by 60% for the high-risk seniors screened as part of the programs.[19]
- Geisinger Health System, Pennsylvania: launched the Fresh Food Farmacy initiative to address food insecurity and to improve patients' diabetes management. The program leverages the health system's electronic health record functionalities and data analytics dashboards to track patients' progress. As of April 2018, the initiative has provided 175,000 meals, decreased the risk of serious complications by more than 40%, and dropped costs by nearly 80% among patients in the pilot program.[20]
- Intermountain Healthcare, Utah: made a $12 million dollar investment that aims to tackle housing instability, utility needs, food insecurity, interpersonal violence, and transportation alongside city, county, and state government agencies and community-based organizations in Utah.
- Kaiser Health, California: implemented the screening tool *Your Current Life Situation*, a survey used in Kaiser's primary care and ED settings. Within the health system's Northwest region, survey responses are included in patients' electronic health records, which are then used by a patient navigator to help them find community resources to meet their social needs. Patient navigators screened 11,273 patients with SDH, identifying and documenting 47,911 SDH in the electronic health record.[21]
- University of Illinois, Illinois: partnered with the Center for Housing and Health to launch the Better Health through Housing initiative in 2015. Under the initiative, hospital providers identified ED patients who were experiencing chronic homelessness and referred them to the community group. The ED reported a 35% reduction in use, and saw participant health care costs fall by 42%, and more recent studies have found that costs have dropped by 61%.[18]
- Nemours Children's Health System, Delaware: created a partnership with Eisenberg Elementary School to convert a classroom into a fully functioning pediatric clinic, complete with doctor's checkups, and mental and behavioral health evaluations. The elementary school is located in a food desert with higher rates of homelessness and a population not plugged in with local pediatricians and significant gaps in their health care. Anticipated outcomes include supplemental medical care that allows children to remain in school and prevent parents from having to miss work.[22]

CASE EXAMPLE
University of Vermont Medical Center: Investments in Social Determinants of Health

The University of Vermont Medical Center (UVMMC) has implemented comprehensive strategies that integrate care coordination strategies with investments in supportive housing. At present, UVMMC has documented savings of $1 million per year because of reduced preventable utilization. Through its participation in the Blueprint for Health, a nationally recognized initiative that designs community-led strategies for improving health and well-being, UVMMC also leads the Accountable Communities for Health in its region to bring together partners from health care, social services, and other sectors to take responsibility for the health of the entire population in a defined geographic area. The model fosters collaboration that engages all the levers of population health—social circumstances, economic conditions, environment, behavior, and more.

In addition as part of the State of Vermont's Blueprint for Health, UVMMC partners with SASH (Support and Services at Home), a statewide model to harnesses the strength of social service agencies, community health providers, and nonprofit housing organizations to support approximately 5000 Vermonters in aging at home. A recent study found that SASH participants demonstrated statistically significant lower growth in expenditure across categories including total Medicare expenditures, emergency room visits, hospital outpatient department visits, and primary care/specialist physician visits. This model was found to decrease growth of Medicare expenses by an estimated $1536 per beneficiary per year.[23]

EDUCATION

In 2016 the Institute of Medicine of the National Academies of Sciences, Engineering, and Medicine convened a committee of experts to develop a high-level framework for incorporating SDH into health professional education resulting in *A Framework for Educating Health Professionals to Address the Social Determinants of Health*. Based on a thorough review of the literature from the study, it was determined that a holistic framework that aligns the education, health, and other sectors, in partnership with communities, to educate health professionals in the SDH is critical for current and future health professionals.[24]

A review of Accreditation Council for Graduate Medical Education residency program requirements also indicates that only family medicine training programs specifically require residents to assess community, environmental, and family influences on health. In recognition of the importance of SDH, the recently implemented Clinical Learning Environment Reviews requires that all residents be involved in addressing health care disparities at the clinical site where they are trained, but do not extend into the community.[25] Improving knowledge, skills, and attitudes around SDH through the use of advanced tools and community-specific learning activities can improve the care of all patients and contribute to addressing SDH as required for success under value-based payment models.

RETURN ON INVESTMENT

Greater attention to SDH can reduce care use patterns, strengthen prevention, and shift services from higher-cost emergency rooms and hospitals to lower-cost primary care settings. Emerging data are starting to quantify the impact of targeting SDH and investing in new care models.

- Researchers from the University of South Florida College of Public Health, Tampa, and WellCare Health Plans found that health care spending is substantially reduced when people are successfully connected to social services that address social barriers. The researchers' study assessed the impact of social services among 2700 Medicaid and Medicare Advantage members on health care costs and reported an additional 10% reduction in health care costs, which equates to more than $2400 per person per year savings for people who were successfully connected to social services compared with a control group of members who were not.[26]

- A 2016 Kaiser Permanente Health Research Initiative report estimated that relying on an extended care team that includes nutritionists, social workers, and community health workers could save providers $1.2 million a year per 10,000 patients in a value-based payment environment.[27]
- The Root Cause Coalition analysis also found that when hospitals and health systems focus their resources on housing supports and case management, net savings can total between $9000 and $30,000 per person per year.[28]

Each example demonstrates the business case for factoring in investments into SDH as part of the overall population health strategy. However, estimating the returns by stakeholder and overall to society can be challenging. The spectrum of benefits range from cost avoidance or savings that result from less tertiary care (eg, lower hospital readmission rates or ED use) to the value of improved health outcomes (such as A1C levels) to the long-term economic impacts, such as worker productivity improvements or lower incarceration rates. It can be difficult to agree not only on what is included in the spectrum of benefits but how to value the more intrinsic outcomes, such as improved quality of life, well-being, and patient experience.[29] The ability to create an agreed-upon methodology that substantiates the cost avoidance and savings of SDH investments is critical to move beyond pilot funding and support more widespread investments in SDH programming.

SUMMARY

In a fee-for-service model, health systems generate more revenue when patient volume increases. Under a value-based model, a person who shows up at an emergency room or a doctor's office becomes an expense rather than a source of revenue. The health care system is shifting toward putting a premium on the quality of care provided as opposed to the number of services provided. With a system that pays for quality and outcomes, physicians must consider the underlying factors that affect a patient's physical health and continued wellness. An increased focus on wellness and prevention presents an opportunity to improve overall population health. One challenge for physicians is the need to develop a broader understanding of how social or environmental determinants may affect a patient's ability to adhere to a care plan. A patient with diabetes who lives in substandard housing, recently lost their job, or lives in a food desert will face greater challenges in managing their illness than a patient who is not facing these obstacles. However, it might not be readily apparent to a physician that a patient living in substandard housing may have trouble keeping their insulin refrigerated because of poor wiring and spotty electricity, or that a patient living in a food desert might also lack reliable transportation options to get to a grocery store with nutritious food. Physicians will be challenged with the need to develop a broader understanding of how social or environmental determinants affect their patient's ability to adhere to a care plan. Although most health systems are still in the early phases of moving toward risk-based reimbursement, a reluctance by health care organizations to assume financial risk for structural factors in the larger economy will inhibit full investment and implementation of SDH models. A 2017 survey on social determinants administered by the health care consulting firm Leavitt Partners asked physicians which factors would "greatly or moderately" benefit their patients.[30] Among the 621 respondents, their answers were:

- Helping patients arrange for transportation (66%)
- Increasing patients' income (54%)
- Helping them get sufficient food (45%)
- Helping them get affordable housing (45%)

From a health system and provider perspective, addressing these determinants as part of a comprehensive strategy is a key to success under value-based payment models because they lead to the Triple Aim of Healthcare—*improved health outcomes, reduced care gaps,* and *financial success.*

The transition to a payment model that rewards value over volume will require a rebalancing of priorities to focus more on preventing or addressing health-damaging social conditions and behavioral choices. Innovations that address SDH are likely to succeed and thrive within a business model, the profit formula of which is rooted in the appropriate form of value-based payments. Reducing the burden of patients' SDH at the individual and population levels also requires a culture of health within communities to develop and maintain strong connections between health care systems, payers, and community-based organizations.[33] Developing successful, efficient approaches to making and maintaining these connections will bolster the ability to address patients' SDH and achieve success under value-based care by reducing the downstream health care use, costs, and health disparities.

REFERENCES

1. Physicians Foundation. 2018 Survey of America's Physicians: practice patterns and perspectives. 2018. Available at: https://www.merritthawkins.com/uploadedFiles/MerrittHawkins/Content/Pdf/MerrittHawkins_PhysiciansFoundation_Survey2018.pdf. Accessed December 30, 2018.
2. World Health Organization. About social determinants of health. 2018. Available at: https://www.who.int/social_determinants/sdh_definition/en/. Accessed December 30, 2018.
3. Office of Health Disease and Promotion. Social determinants of health. 2018. Available at: https://www.healthypeople.gov/2020/topics-objectives/topic/social-determinants-of-health. Accessed December 30, 2018.
4. Anderson C, Squires D. US healthcare from a global perspective: spending, use of services and health in 13 countries. Commonwealth Fund; 2015. Available at: https://www.commonwealthfund.org/publications/issue-briefs/2015/oct/us-health-care-global-perspective. Accessed December 30, 2018.
5. Bresnick J. AMIA: consider broadband access a social determinant of health. Health IT Analytics. 2017. Available at: https://healthitanalytics.com/news/amia-consider-broadband-access-a-social-determinate-of-health. Accessed December 30, 2018.
6. Fenton J. Health care's blind side. Robert Wood Johnson Foundation; 2011. Available at: https://www.rwjf.org/en/library/research/2011/12/health-care-s-blind-side.html. Accessed December 30, 2018.
7. Robert Wood Johnson Foundation. Could where you are born influence where you live?. 2018. Available at: https://www.rwjf.org/en/library/interactives/whereyouliveaffectshowlongyoulive.html. Accessed December 30, 2018.
8. American Hospital Association. Addressing social determinants of health presentation. 2018. Available at: https://www.aha.org/addressing-social-determinants-health-presentation. Accessed December 30, 2018.

9. Center for Medicaid and Medicare Services. CMS proposes to modernize Medicare advantage, expand telehealth access for patients. CMS.gov Newsroom. 2018. Available at: https://www.cms.gov/newsroom/press-releases/cms-proposes-modernize-medicare-advantage-expand-telehealth-access-patients. Accessed December 30, 2018.

10. Kung K, Zablocki A. Medicare advantage to address social determinants of health: an important step for value-based care. SherpardMullin healthcare blog. 2018. Available at: https://www.sheppardhealthlaw.com/2018/04/articles/medicare/medicare-advantage/sdoh-value-based-care/. Accessed December 30, 2018.

11. Beaton T. 80% of payers aim to address social determinants of health. Health payer intelligence. 2018. Available at: https://healthpayerintelligence.com/news/80-of-payers-aim-to-address-social-determinants-of-health. Accessed December 30, 2018.

12. Machledt D. Addressing the social determinants of health through Medicaid managed care. The Commonwealth Fund; 2017. Available at: https://www.commonwealthfund.org/publications/issue-briefs/2017/nov/addressing-social-determinants-health-through-medicaid-managed. Accessed December 30, 2018.

13. Antonisse L, Edwards BC, Ellis E, et al. States focus on quality and outcomes amid waiver changes: results from a 50-state Medicaid budget survey for state fiscal years 2018 and 2019. Kaiser Family Foundation; 2018. Available at: https://www.kff.org/report-section/states-focus-on-quality-and-outcomes-amid-waiver-changes-managed-care-initiatives/. Accessed December 30, 2018.

14. LaForge K, Gold R, Cottrell E, et al. How 6 organizations developed tools and processes for social determinants of health screening in primary care: an overview. J Ambul Care Manage 2017;41(1):2–14.

15. Thomas-Henkel C, Schulman M. Screening for social determinants of health in populations with complex needs: implementation considerations. Center for Healthcare Strategies Inc; 2017. Available at: https://www.chcs.org/media/SDOH-Complex-Care-Screening-Brief-102617.pdf. Accessed December 30, 2018.

16. Center for Medicare and Medicaid Services. Accountable health communities model. 2018. Available at: https://innovation.cms.gov/initiatives/ahcm/. Accessed December 30, 2018.

17. Korba C, Lee J. Social determinants of health: how are hospitals and health systems investing in social needs? Deloitte Center for Health Solutions. 2017. Available at: https://www2.deloitte.com/us/en/pages/life-sciences-and-health-care/articles/addressing-social-determinants-of-health-hospitals-survey.html. Accessed December 30, 2018.

18. LaPointe J. Revcycle intelligence. Retrieved from: how addressing social determinants of health cuts healthcare costs. 2018. Available at: https://revcycleintelligence.com/news/how-addressing-social-determinants-of-health-cuts-healthcare-costs. Accessed December 30, 2018.

19. Johnson S. Complete care: hospitals tackling social determinants set the course. Modern Healthcare. 2017. Available at: https://www.modernhealthcare.com/article/20180825/NEWS/180809949. Accessed December 30, 2018.

20. Coolbaugh S, Feinberg A, Hess A, et al. Prescribing food as a specialty drug. NEJM catalyst. 2018. Available at: https://catalyst.nejm.org/prescribing-fresh-food-farmacy/. Accessed December 30, 2018.

21. Friedman NL, Banegas MP. Toward addressing social determinants of health: a health care system strategy. Perm J 2018;22:18–095.

22. Heath S. As connected health use grows, value-based care models must follow. Patient engagement HIT. 2018. Available at: https://patientengagementhit.com/news/as-connected-health-use-grows-value-based-care-models-must-follow. Accessed December 30, 2018.

23. Edwards P, Eicheldinger C, Kandilov A, et al. Support and Services at Home (SASH) evaluation: second annual report. Washington DC: US Department of Health and Human Services- Office of the Assistant Secretary for Planning and Evaluation; 2016. Available at: https://aspe.hhs.gov/basic-report/support-and-services-home-sash-evaluation-second-annual-report. Accessed December 30, 2018.

24. National Academies of Sciences, Engineering, and Medicine. A framework for educating health professionals to address the social determinants of health. Washington, DC: The National Academies Press; 2016.

25. Clements DS. Social determinants of health in family residency education. Ann Fam Med 2018;16:178.

26. Landi H. Study: addressing patients' social barriers reduces healthcare spending. Healthcare informatics. 2018. Available at: https://www.healthcare-informatics.com/news-item/population-health/study-addressing-patients-social-determinants-health-reduces-healthcare. Accessed December 30, 2018.

27. PWC Research Institute. Top health industries issues of 2018: a year for resilience amid uncertainty. 2018. Available at: https://www.kpcareerplanning.org/prd/include/pwc-health-research-institute-top-health-industry-issues-of-2018-report.pdf. Accessed December 30, 2018.

28. The root cause coalition. Housing and health: the connection and innovative steps health systems are taking to address housing to improve health. 2016. Available at: http://www.rootcausecoalition.org/wp-content/uploads/2016/11/White-Paper-Housing-and-Health.pdf. Accessed December 30, 2018.

29. Altarum Healthcare Hub. Tapping into the benefits of social investments: addressing financing silos. 2018. Available at: https://www.healthcarevaluehub.org/advocate-resources/publications/tapping-benefits-social-investments-addressing-financing-silos/; https://www.advisory.com/daily-briefing/2018/05/15/social-determinants. Accessed December 30, 2018.

30. Institute of Medicine (US) Committee on assuring the health of the public in the 21st century. The future of the public's health in the 21st century. Understanding population health and its determinants. Washington (DC): National Academies Press (US); 2002. p. 2. Available at: https://www.ncbi.nlm.nih.gov/books/NBK221225/. Accessed December 30, 2018.

Public Policy Approaches to Population Health

Adam J. Zolotor, MD, DrPH*, Berkeley Yorkery, MPP

KEYWORDS

- Population health • Public health • Public policy • Access • Aging • Early childhood
- Mental health • Opioids

KEY POINTS

- Health policy can have profound effects on health at the federal, state, and local levels.
- Access to health care historically underpins much of the health policy debate in the United States. Programs, such as Medicare, Medicaid, military benefits, and the Affordable Care Act, have been fundamental to increasing access to health insurance and thus health care.
- Early childhood influences health through the life course. Starting children off on the right track has lifelong returns.
- Key to addressing the aging baby boomers will be a high-functioning and adequately funded system of home-based and community-based services.
- Much of the health policy emphasis on opioids to date has focused on prescribing. Policy makers must look beyond supply and address the challenges that create addiction in communities.

INTRODUCTION

The United States currently spends 17.8% of the gross domestic product (GDP) on health care and is on track to spend 19.9% of GDP on health care by 2025—vastly more than any nation in its economic peer group.[1] And for this massive investment, the United States has the highest rate of infant mortality, the lowest life expectancy at birth, the highest rates of obesity, and the largest percent of the over-65-year-old population with 2 or more chronic conditions (compared with countries in its economic peer group). Although the United States spends the most on health care of nations in its economic peer group, the total spending on health and social care combined is actually similar. Most other developed economies spend far less on health and far more on social care, including safety net programs, education, food, housing, and work training.[2]

Disclosure Statement: The authors have nothing to disclose.
North Carolina Institute of Medicine, 630 Davis Drive, Suite 100, Morrisville, NC 27560, USA
* Corresponding author.
E-mail address: Adam_Zolotor@nciom.org

Public policy sets a foundation for much of the work of population health. Although population health may be influenced by private and nonprofit entities, including health systems, insurers, and nongovernmental organizations, the public sector funds the vast majority of population health efforts in the United States and creates a regulatory environment in which the work of population health improvement is carried out.

Policy levers that affect population health most commonly are discussed in the federal and state contexts. The policy opportunities that exist in counties, municipalities, and school districts, however, should be kept in mind. One of the most important policy levers to have implications on population health is simply the budget (federal, state, and county). The vast sums of money used for public insurance programs (Medicare, Medicaid, military and veteran insurance, and marketplace subsidies) have a profound impact on access to care. Within and outside of the purse authority, federal and state governments use policy to create incentives to improve quality, limit or enhance reimbursement to incentivize certain types of services, and regulate the type of coverage and rules around coverage to balance the needs to the purchaser (often the employer) and the beneficiary of health care.

Beyond access to health care, policy makers have purview over a great many policy levers to influence population health. Policy strategies include funding of direct services with a clear link to health (such as supplemental nutrition programs) and those that are critical for health but with a less direct link (such as housing and transportation programs). Policy makers have purview over product labeling regulations, clean air and water, the development of transportation infrastructure (including greenways), the farm bill (and resultant flooding of food supply with processed corn products), and the federal school nutrition program.

Some important areas of state authority include design and eligibility for Medicaid, joint funding and required state match for a broad array of community services, funding for school nurses, behavioral health services for those without insurance, and the design and enforcement of a vast array of laws to make streets and neighborhoods safer (such as speed limits and enforcement, seatbelt laws, and community violence prevention programs). At the levels of county and municipal government, health officials have authority for community health and assessment, planning, and public health enforcement.

The lines between federal, state, and local government authorities to influence population health are frequently gray, often due to shared responsibility. The largest investment by far in efforts to improve population health is made by the federal government. State and local policy makers, however, exert influence through state and local funding match, knowledge of state and local conditions and relationships with constituents, and implementation of programs and policies.

ACCESS

Access to high-quality health care is important for promoting and maintaining health, preventing and managing disease, and achieving health equity.[3] Whether individuals have access to care is determined by many factors, including the ability to afford care, the availability of care, and whether the individuals can find a provider they trust and with whom they can communicate. Health insurance coverage is the most significant factor in whether health care is affordable. In the United States, there is no single system for health insurance coverage. In 2017, approximately 56% of US residents had private health insurance, 36% relied on public health insurance, and 9% were uninsured.[4]

Private Health Insurance

Private health insurance refers to insurance that is not administered by federal, state, or local government. Most people with private health insurance (88%) are enrolled in employer-based coverage, meaning they (and often their families) gain access to and purchase their health insurance through their employer.[5] The cost of employer-based coverage varies widely because there are a range of cost-sharing agreements between employers and employees. A small percentage (12%) of those in the private health insurance market purchase their own health insurance through either the health insurance marketplaces established by the Affordable Care Act (ACA) or outside the marketplaces. ACA plans are subject to federal requirements for which benefits are covered and cost-sharing levels and cannot exclude individuals due to preexisting conditions. Non-ACA plans do not have to meet these requirements.

Public Health Insurance

Public health insurance refers to insurance programs run by federal, state, or local government, including Medicare, Medicaid, and Tricare and Veterans Affairs (VA) health care. Medicare is the federal health insurance program that covers individuals 65 years and older as well as some permanently disabled individuals under age 65.[6] Although often portrayed as a uniform program, Medicare has multiple parts (A, B, C, D, and supplemental coverage) that are provided by either Medicare or private insurance companies approved by Medicare and that vary in coverage and cost.

- Part A (traditional Medicare): hospital insurance provided by Medicare
- Part B (traditional Medicare): medical insurance provided by Medicare
- Part C (Medicare Advantage): hospital and medical insurance provided by private insurance companies
- Part D: prescription drug coverage provided by private insurance companies (typically already included in Part C plans)
- Supplemental coverage (Medigap): health care costs that are not covered by Parts A and B, such as copayments, coinsurance, and deductibles

Medicare does not cover all services, notably long-term care services.

Medicaid is a program funded jointly by federal and state government that is administered by states. The percentage of the program funded by the federal government, the Federal Medical Assistance Percentage, varies by state, with the federal government covering between 50% and 76% of the cost of Medicaid.[7] States establish and administer their own Medicaid programs within the federal guidelines. This state-by-state system results in wide variations in the type, amount, duration, and scope of services covered.[8] Medicaid benefit coverage also varies by state but generally covers low-income individuals, including children, pregnant women, seniors, and people with disabilities.[9] Most states contract with managed care organizations for the delivery of services to Medicaid beneficiaries.[10] Tricare and VA health care are federal programs to meet the needs of US service members, retirees, and their families.

Individuals Without Insurance

Individuals who do not have health insurance face significant challenges to accessing health care. They are more likely to forego needed health care because of costs, to report being in fair or poor health, to be hospitalized for preventable conditions, to have outstanding medical bills, and to die prematurely.[11–13] Individuals without health insurance may be able to receive care through a safety net provider. Safety net providers are those who deliver a significant level of health care services to the uninsured and other vulnerable populations. There are many types of safety net providers (eg, Federally Qualified Health Centers, rural health clinics, free and charitable clinics, local health departments, hospitals, and others) who may, depending on resources, be able to help meet the health needs of the individuals who do not have health insurance.

The Impact of the Affordable Care Act

Discussion of access to health care in the United States now largely focuses on the ACA, passed in 2010. The ACA had ramifications for all aspects of health care. Most ongoing debates, however, are around Medicaid expansion and affordable health insurance. Under the ACA, states have the option to expand Medicaid eligibility up to 138% of the federal poverty line for all residents, which significantly expands coverage. As of September 2019, all but 14 states, mostly in the south, have expanded Medicaid eligibility under the ACA. News coverage about the ACA is dominated by debates around subsidies, insurance rate increases, availability of coverage, and other issues that have an impact on individual plans sold through the health insurance marketplace.

EARLY CHILDHOOD

The health status of young children has a significant impact on the trajectory of their health during adolescence and into adulthood. Children with good health and a strong sense of well-being are more likely to grow into adaptable, functioning adults equipped with the kinds of skills needed to contribute positively to their communities.[14] For this reason, early childhood often is a focus of population health work.

Adverse Childhood Experiences

Significant adversity early in life—such as persistent poverty, exposure to violence, a parent with mental health and/or substance abuse disorders, and poor child care conditions—leads to high levels of stress and negative short-term and long-term outcomes. Research shows that adverse experiences during childhood, such as psychological, physical, or sexual abuse and living with household members who have substance abuse or mental health disorders, are strongly associated with long-term health risk behaviors, health status, and even adult diseases.[15] Adverse childhood experiences are linked to heart disease, obesity, lung disease, diabetes, depression, anxiety, and substance addiction in adulthood. Research shows that warm, stable, loving relationships with caregivers and exposure to high-quality, safe environments can help mitigate the risks associated with adverse childhood experiences.[16]

Early Childhood Mental Health

The mental health of a young child is the achievement of expected developmental cognitive, social, and emotional milestones.[17] Young children's mental health, or social-emotional health, affects how they relate to and interact with others, how they learn, and how well they are able to manage their emotions. The primary social-emotional milestones during the first 5 years of life include developing trusting relationships with caregivers, the ability to signal needs, the full range of feelings and emotions, self-regulation of biological needs, strategies for dealing with separation, and the capacity for social interaction with peers and exploring the environment.[18] Young child mental health influences every single critical developmental task of the first 5 years, whether physical, cognitive, or social-emotional. When left untreated, the presence of mental health problems in young children foretells an ongoing need for costly services later in life.

Early Childhood Programs, Policies, and Services

For young children, the quality and reliability of relationships with their caregivers, the quality and safety of their environment, and the quality of their nutrition form the basic foundation on which child health—physical, mental, and social-emotional well-being—are built.[19] There are many ways to support positive early child development, including programs, policies, and services to

- Strengthen the relationships young children have with their caregivers
  - Parenting programs
  - Early care and education teacher competencies standards
- Improve the environments of young children
  - Subsidies for high-quality child care
  - Head Start and Early Head Start
  - State standards for early care and education settings
- Improve early childhood nutrition
  - Special Supplemental Nutrition Program for Women, Infants, and Children
  - Early care and education food standards
- Teach young children social and emotional skills and
  - Training of early care and education teachers
  - Implementing curriculum standards that include social and emotional learning
- Provide treatment of young children and their families
  - Early intervention services
  - Training programs for primary care and mental health professionals who work for young children

Such strategies positively shape and strengthen young children's environments as well as provide services and supports to address the developmental needs of young children and their families.[19]

AGING

The so-called Silver Tsunami will have profound effects on the cost and delivery of care over the next several decades. This challenge is caused by the aging of baby boomers, or those born between 1946 and 1964 during an increase in birth rate as soldiers returned home from World War II, and the increase in life expectancy over the past century. In 2016, 15.2% of Americans were 65 years and older (49 million). By 2030, the year all baby boomers will be 65 years and over, this proportion will be 20.6% (73 million). At the same time, the population ages 85 years and over will increase by approximately 50% and the 100 years and older population will increase by 70%.[20] Significant increases in the older adult population present a challenge due to the increase in chronic conditions, physical and mental limitations that impair functioning, and social isolation. The challenge of population health for older Americans is further compounded by the decreasing number of adult caretakers who will be available to care for elders in the next decade. This phenomenon, sometimes known as the baby bust, occurred as the birth rate plummeted after the baby boom. The result is that in 2030, there will be half as many adults in middle age (40–65 years) for every 1 older adult (over 80) as there were in 2010.[21] This deficit will create a rapidly increasing strain on the physical, mental, and financial health of those caretakers as well as the system of care and payment for long-term care for older Americans. Caring for the aging population will require innovative approaches to caretaking, housing, and health care. Enough nursing homes to care for this population as it grows (and potential adult caretakers shrink) simply cannot be built. And even if they could be, paying for this care would be an enormous burden.

The current average cost of nursing home care is $92,376 per year, a formidable cost for most Americans.[22] So, who will pay for this care? Medicare pays for a relatively small portion of nursing home stays, limited to up to 100 days after an acute hospitalization. A meager 7.2 million Americans have long-term care insurance and only 11% of those over age 65.[23] Medicaid is the primary payer for long-term care, approximately $55 billion in 2015.[24] This price tag represents a dramatic potential cost to state budgets—given the federal/state match for the payment of Medicaid services. Eligibility criteria for Medicaid coverage for long-term services and support varies by state, but beneficiaries must meet categorical and financial requirements.[25] The portion of nursing home residents whose care is paid for by Medicaid is 62%, an approximately 30% increase since 1977.[24,26]

States and the federal government need to be increasingly innovative in the provision and payment of services, with a focus on keeping people in their homes and communities as long as possible. Three important levers are the move to value in Medicare, alternate payment models or waivers in Medicaid, and direct payment for home-based and community-based services not tied to insurance.

Increasingly, Medicare beneficiaries are signing up for Medicare managed care plans or Medicare Advantage plans, rather than the traditional Medicare.[27] These plans may appeal to consumers because of array of services, copays, and premiums. Consumers should be cautious in shopping among these plans, because cost savings can be created through narrow networks and limited formularies. These plans may use flexibility created by fee-for-value arrangements, however, such as quality incentives to provide community services.

Medicaid waiver programs for the elderly and disabled are critical means by which to support people in their homes and communities. These programs, known collectively as Medicaid Home- and Community-Based Services, include the 1915(c) waiver services, personal care state plan services, and home health state plan services. On these types of services, Medicaid collective spent nearly $61 billion in 2014.[28] A majority of enrollees and expenditures are in the 1915(c) programs. These programs represent an extensive array of services designed to maximize the quality of life and functional status of beneficiaries in their homes and have an average cost of $26,563 per year per beneficiary. These programs often result in an upfront increase in cost but save money in the long run because people remain in their homes longer, forestalling or avoiding costly nursing home care.[29] Many such programs have long waiting lists. It also is important to underscore that these services are only for Medicaid beneficiaries or those of low income and low wealth.

In addition to Medicare and Medicaid programs to pay for home-based and community-based services, there is an array of services paid for by federal funds (through the home-based and community-based services block grant) and individual state programs. These programs typically use income eligibility guidelines and may include medical transportation, home delivered meals, respite services, and adult day care, among other services. These services also often have waiting lists and, in most cases, serve people below or near the poverty level.[30]

MENTAL HEALTH

Mental health and substance use disorders are common, with 1 in 6 adults in the United States having had any mental illness in the past year and 1 in 12 ages 12 and older having a substance use disorder.[31] Although some mental health and substance use disorders are precipitated in response to disruptive life events, most are chronic or recurrent conditions that, like other chronic illnesses, require ongoing care and treatment. As with any chronic disease, prevention, identification, treatment, and recovery services and supports are essential to ensuring positive health outcomes. Prevention, treatment, and recovery services and supports are essential to ensuring positive health outcomes for people with mental health and substance use disorders. These services, when managed and implemented effectively, can minimize long-term costs to individuals, families, businesses, and governments.[31]

Coverage Barriers

Although 2 federal laws, the Paul Wellstone and Pete Domenici Mental Health Parity and Addiction Equity Act of 2008 and the ACA, greatly expanded coverage by requiring most insurance plans to cover mental health and substance use services at parity with medical and surgical benefits, many with health insurance still struggle to access mental health and substance use services. Insurance coverage still varies significantly on the kinds of services, quantity of services, and the types of professionals covered as well as the authorization processes required to access various services. Additionally, many individuals with mental health and substance use needs are uninsured.[32,33] There is little funding for services for the uninsured.

Fragmentated Systems

In addition to coverage barriers, individuals face barriers to receiving needed prevention, treatment, and recovery services, contributing to unnecessary and avoidable disability, school failure, homelessness, and incarceration.[34] A significant challenge is that there is no single system for mental health and substance use services, making access to services particularly difficult for individuals. The system includes a variety of fragmented providers and services and the various agencies that provide funding and oversight.

Other Barriers

Access to mental health and substance use services varies significantly by geographic location, with access better in urban areas than rural ones. Access to appropriate services is also impacted by type of mental health or substance use disorder and age. Additionally, strong cultural stigmas against seeking out mental health treatment still exist and affect utilization of services.

Programs, Policies, and Services to Improve Access to Mental Health Services

On average, individuals with severe mental illness die earlier than those in the general population, mainly due to overlooked or poorly managed physical health conditions.[35] Although individuals' mental health and physical health are inextricably intertwined, the US medical system historically has had different models of care for mental health and physical health needs. This division has created barriers for individuals with both mental health and physical health needs. Integrated care, the systematic coordination of physical and mental health care, is an evidence-based, effective approach.[36] Transforming practices from traditional medical/mental health and substance use practices into integrated care practices, however, often requires substantial technical assistance.

There is a shortage of mental health and substance use professionals in many communities. One way to mitigate this shortage is to provide services for individuals with mental health and substance use disorders remotely using technology. Telebehavioral health focuses on mental health and substance use outcomes, and studies have shown its success in improving consumer well-being. Telepsychiatry also is cost-effective.[37–39] Challenges to implementing telemedicine mental health and substance use models include the need to provide reliable Internet connectivity, videoconferencing equipment to providers, and health insurance integration.

OPIOIDS

The past 2 decades have seen a rapid rise in opioid use, addiction, and fatality, with more than 400,000 opioid overdose deaths since 1999. There are many reasons for this epidemic. Addiction was common in the decades that preceded the opioid epidemic but often to much less lethal drugs. In the 1990s, health care providers were implored to treat pain, pain was measured as the fifth vital sign, and the pharmaceutical industry embarked on a massive marketing campaign to convince health care providers and the public that these drugs were much less addictive than they really are. What followed was a massive increase in the availability of these highly addictive and much more lethal drugs.

Policy makers have largely focused on ways to control prescribing as a way to address the supply of these drugs. Federal guidelines, state medical board policy, the development of infrastructure (such as prescription drug monitoring programs), and more recently legal mandates and limited prescribing have all been deployed to address this epidemic. These efforts have resulted in a modest decrease in prescribing—13% from 2010 to 2015.[40] But Americans are still prescribed 60% more opioids than Canadians and approximately 400% more than people in most European countries.[41] Despite efforts to curtail prescribing and widespread distribution of naloxone (opioid reversal drug), opioid overdose deaths are at an all-time high, up 9.6% from 2016 to 2017.[42] Additionally, evidence has shown that as opioid prescribing declines, reducing access to opioids in communities, the use of heroin and other highly potent synthetic opioids increases.

There are numerous other policy levers to combat the opioid epidemic, but most will require new resources and political will. New harm-reduction strategies, such as supervised use centers; increased investment in treatment, including medication-assisted therapies; adequate alternatives to treating acute and chronic pain; investments in law enforcement strategies to curb illegal sales; and, ultimately, addressing the conditions that are the root cause of addiction, such as community despair, poverty, and violence.

SUMMARY

Policy makers have significant influence over population health not only through the power of the purse and as a result of taxation but also by the development and implementation of regulations and programs. Many in health care live with the benefits and consequences of these policies as patients are cared for. Why are poor adults not Medicaid eligible in my state (failure to expand Medicaid under the ACA)? Why must I stop each time I want to prescribe an opiate and check the prescription drug monitoring program (state laws vary, but many now require this every 3 months)? Why am I penalized financially when my patients do not show up for their appointments (variety of federal and state laws that require quality reporting for Medicaid and Medicare as well as the private insurance regulatory market)? Although these represent only a few of the barriers that health care providers face in working with patients, they highlight the larger role that policy plays in the lives of all people.

Federal, state, and local systems and policies shape the conditions in which individuals live, work, learn, and age. In other words, policy makers influence almost every aspect of population health. It is critical that health care providers and their institutions and associations remain informed and engaged in the policy making process.

REFERENCES

1. Keehan SP, Stone DA, Poisal JA, et al. National health expenditure projections, 2016-25: price increases, aging push sector to 20 percent of economy. Health Aff (Millwood) 2017;36(3):553–63.
2. Squires D. U.S. Health care from a global perspective spending, use of services, prices, and health in 13 countries. New York 2018. Available at: https://www. commonwealthfund.org/publications/issue-briefs/2015/oct/us-health-care-global-perspective. Accessed January 10, 2019.
3. US Department of Health and Human Services. Healthy people 2020: access to health services. Washington, DC: Office of Disease Prevention and Health Promotion; 2019. Available at: https://www.healthypeople.gov/2020/topics-objectives/topic/Access-to-Health-Services. Accessed January 10, 2019.
4. Kaiser Family Foundation. Health insurance coverage of the total population, 2017 2019. San Francisco, CA. Available at: https://www.kff.org/other/state-indicator/total-population/?dataView=1&currentTimeframe=0&sortModel=%7B%22colId%22:%22Location%22,%22sort%22:%22desc%22%7D. Accessed January 10, 2019.
5. NCIOM. Claims data to improve health in North Carolina: a report from the NCIOM task force on all payer claims database. Morrisville, NC 2017. Available at: http://nciom.org/apcd/. Accessed January 10, 2019.
6. Centers for Medicare and Medicaid Services. Medicare Program- General Information. Baltimore, MD: US Department of Health and Human Services. Available at: https://www.cms.gov/Medicare/Medicare-General-Information/MedicareGenInfo/index.html. Accessed January 11, 2019.
7. US Department of Health and Human Services. Federal matching shares for Medicaid, the children's health insurance program, and aid to needy aged, blind or disabled persons for October 1, 2018 through September 30 2019. Washington, DC. Available at: https://www.federalregister.gov/documents/2017/11/21/2017-24953/federal-matching-shares-for-medicaid-the-childrens-health-insurance-program-and-aid-to-needy-aged. Accessed January 10, 2019.
8. Centers for Medicare and Medicaid Services. Medicaid program: benefits. Baltimore, MD: US Department of Health and Human Services. Available at: https://www.medicaid.gov/medicaid/benefits/index.html. Accessed January 10, 2019.
9. Medicaid. Medicaid Eligibility. Baltimore, MD. Available at: https://www.medicaid.gov/medicaid/eligibility/index.html. Accessed January 11, 2019.
10. Kaiser Family Foundation. Total Medicaid MCOs. San Francisco, CA. Available at: https://www.kff.org/medicaid/state-indicator/total-medicaid-mcos/?currentTimeframe=0&sortModel=%7B%22colId%22:%22Location%22,%22sort%22:%22asc%22%7D. Accessed January 10, 2019.
11. Kaiser Family Foundation. The uninsured: a primer. Key Facts about Americans without health insurance. San Francisco, CA 2012. Available at: https://

kaiserfamilyfoundation.files.wordpress.com/2013/01/7451-08.pdf. Accessed March 13, 2019.

12. Simon K, Soni A, Cawley J. The impact of health insurance on preventive care and health behaviors: evidence from the first two years of the ACA medicaid expansions. J Policy Anal Manage 2017;36(2):390–417.

13. Wherry LR, Miller S. Early coverage, access, utilization, and health effects associated with the affordable care act medicaid expansions: a quasi-experimental Study. Ann Intern Med 2016;164(12):795–803.

14. Miles J, Espiritu RC, Horen NM, et al. A public health approach to children's mental health a conceptual framework. Washington, DC: Georgetown University Center for Child and Human Development, National Technical Assistance Center for Children's Mental Health; 2010. Available at: http://gucchdtacenter.georgetown.edu/publications/PublicHealthApproach.pdf?CFID=4150182&CFTOKEN=89131034. Accessed January 10, 2019.

15. National Center for Chronic Disease Prevention and Health Promotion. Adverse childhood experiences (ACE) study. Atlanta, GA: Centers for Disease Control and Prevention; 2010. Available at: http://www.cdc.gov/ace/prevalence.htm. Accessed January 10, 2019.

16. National Scientific Council on the Developing Child. Excessive stress disrupts the architecture of the developing brain. Working Paper No. 3 2004. Cambridge, MA. Available at: http://www.developingchild.net. Accessed January 10, 2019.

17. US Department of Health and Human Services. Substance abuse and mental health administration. Mental health: a report of the surgeon general. Rockville, MD 1999. Available at: http://profiles.nlm.nih.gov/ps/access/NNBBHS.pdf. Accessed January 10, 2019.

18. Johnson MR, Appleyard K. Infant psychosocial disorders. In: Bremner JG, Wachs TD, editors. Wiley-Blackwell Handbook of infant development, vol. 2, 2nd edition. Oxford (UK): Wiley-Blackwell; 2010. p. 280–307.

19. Center for the Developing Child. The foundations of lifelong health are built in early childhood. Cambridge, MA 2010. Available at: www.developingchild.harvard.edu. Accessed January 10, 2019.

20. US Census Bureau. An aging nation: projected number of children and older adults. Washington, DC 2018. Available at: https://www.census.gov/library/visualizations/2018/comm/historic-first.html. Accessed January 10, 2019.

21. Redfoot D, Feinberg L, Houser A. Baby boom and the growing care gap: a look at future declines in The … AARP Public Policy Institute. Washington, DC. Available at: http://www.aarp.org/home-family/caregiving/info-08-2013/the-aging-of-the-baby-boom-and-the-growing-care-gap-AARP-ppi-ltc.html. Accessed January 11, 2019.

22. Senior living. Nursing home costs in 2019 by state and type of care. Available at: SeniorLiving.org https://www.seniorliving.org/lifestyles/nursing-homes/costs/. Accessed January 11, 2019.

23. Gleckman H. Who owns long-term care insurance? Forbes 2016. New jersey. Available at: https://www.forbes.com/sites/howardgleckman/2016/08/18/who-owns-long-term-care-insurance/#33813fe92f05. Accessed January 11, 2019.

24. Kaiser Family Foundation. Medicaid's role in nursing home care 2017. San Francisco, CA. Available at: https://www.kff.org/infographic/medicaids-role-in-nursing-home-care/. Accessed January 11, 2019.

25. Congressional Research Service. Medicaid financial eligibility for long-term services and supports. Washington, DC 2017. Available at: https://fas.org/sgp/crs/misc/R43506.pdf. Accessed January 10, 2019.

26. Ness J, Ahmed A, Aronow WS. Demographics and payment characteristics of nursing home residents in the United States: a 23-year trend. J Gerontol A Biol Sci Med Sci 2004;59(11):1213–7.

27. Jacobson G, Damico A, Neuman T. Medicare advantage 2017 spotlight: enrollment market update. San Francisco, CA: Kaiser Family Foudation; 2017. Available at: https://www.kff.org/medicare/issue-brief/medicare-advantage-2017-spotlight-enrollment-market-update/. Accessed January 11, 2019.

28. Watts MO. Medicaid home and community-based services: results from a 50-state survey of enrollment, spending, and program policies 2018. San Francisco, CA. Available at: https://www.kff.org/report-section/medicaid-home-and-community-based-services-results-trom-a-50-state-survoy-of-enrollment-spending-and-program-policies-report/. Accessed January 11, 2019.

29. Fox-Grage W, Walls J. State studies find home and community-based services to be cost effective. Washington, DC: AARP Public Policy Institute; 2013. Available at: https://www.aarp.org/health/medicare-insurance/info-03-2013/state-studies-find-hcbs-to-be-cost-effective-AARP-ppi-ltc.html. Accessed January 11, 2019.

30. NCIOM. Dementia-capable North Carolina: a strategic plan for addressing alzheimer's disease and related dementias. Morrisville, NC: NCIOM; 2016. Available at: http://nciom.org/dementia-capable-north-carolina-a-strategic-plan-for-addressing-alzheimers-disease-and-related-dementias/. Accessed January 11, 2019.

31. Substance Abuse and mental Health Services Administration. Key Substance Use and Mental Health Indicators in the United States: Results from the 2016 National Survey on Drug Use and Health (HHS Publication No. SMA 17-5044, NSDUH Series H-52. Center for Behavioral Health Statistics and Quality, Substance Abuse and Mental Health Services Administration. Washington, DC. Available at: https://www.samhsa.gov/data/sites/default/files/NSDUH-FFR1-2016/NSDUH-FFR1-2016.pdf. Accessed January 10, 2019.

32. Substance Abuse and Mental Health Services Administration. Health insurance status of adult substance abuse treatment admissions aged 26 or older: 2011. Washington, DC 2014. Available at: https://www.samhsa.gov/data/sites/default/files/sr134-health-insurance-2014/sr134-health-insurance-2014/sr134-health-insurance-2014.htm. Accessed January 10, 2019.

33. Mental Health America. Mental Health in America - Access to Care Data. Alexandria, VA. Available at: http://www.mentalhealthamerica.net/issues/mental-health-america-access-care-data. Accessed January 10, 2019.

34. NCIOM. Transforming North Carolina's mental health and substance use systems: a report from the NCIOM task force on mental health and substance use. Morrisville, NC 2015. Available at: http://nciom.org/transforming-north-carolinas-mental-health-and-substance-use-systems-a-report-from-the-nciom-task-force-on-mental-health-and-substance-use/. Accessed January 11, 2019.

35. World Health Organization. Premature death among people with severe mental disorders. Geneva, Switzerland. Available at: https://www.who.int/mental_health/management/info_sheet.pdf. Accessed January 10, 2019.

36. Substance Abuse and Mental Health Services Administration. What is integrated care? Washington, DC. Available at: https://www.integration.samhsa.gov/about-us/what-is-integrated-care. Accessed January 10, 2019.

37. Ruskin PE, Silver-Aylaian M, Kling MA, et al. Treatment outcomes in depression: comparison of remote treatment through telepsychiatry to in-person treatment. Am J Psychiatry 2004;161(8):1471–6.

38. Nobis S, Ebert DD, Lehr D, et al. Web-based intervention for depressive symptoms in adults with types 1 and 2 diabetes mellitus: a health economic evaluation. Br J Psychiatry 2018;212(4):199–206.
39. Hyler SE, Gangure DP. A review of the costs of telepsychiatry. Psychiatr Serv 2003;54(7):976–80.
40. Guy GP, Zhang K, Bohm MK, et al. Vital Signs: changes in opioid prescribing in the United States, 2006-2015. MMWR Morb Mortal Wkly Rep 2017;66(26): 697–704.
41. International Narcotics Control Board. Narcotic drugs-technical report. New York: United Nations; 2018. Available at: https://www.incb.org/incb/en/narcotic-drugs/ Technical_Reports/narcotic_drugs_reports.html. Accessed January 11, 2019.
42. Centers for Disease Control and Prevention. Drug overdose deaths 2018. Atlanta, GA. Available at: https://www.cdc.gov/drugoverdose/data/statedeaths.html. Accessed January 11, 2019.

Community and Stakeholder Engagement

Mina Silberberg, PhD[a],*, Viviana Martinez-Bianchi, MD[b]

KEYWORDS

- Population health • Stakeholder engagement • Community engagement
- Principles of engagement

KEY POINTS

- Improving population health in a sustainable way requires working through partnerships among multiple community and societal stakeholders.
- One particularly important form of stakeholder engagement is engagement of the community whose health will be directly affected, often referred to as community engagement.
- Stakeholder engagement has multiple benefits for the quality, sustainability, and impact of population health research and interventions.
- Several principles of engagement have been developed; common elements are power sharing, respect, humility, colearning, commitment, and a goal of making change.
- There is an ever-widening pool of resources available to help clinicians who wish to enhance their skills in stakeholder engagement.

WHAT IS STAKEHOLDER ENGAGEMENT? WHY DOES IT MATTER?

Population health refers to sustainable pragmatic efforts to improve health and health equity through attention to population-level determinants of health. Because lifestyles, behaviors, and the incidence of illness are all shaped by social and physical environments, improving population health in a sustainable way requires working through partnerships among multiple community and societal stakeholders.[1,2] Health issues are best addressed by engaging partners who can bring to a project the diverse relevant perspectives, understandings, and resources. Depending on the nature of the issue and the social and political dynamics surrounding it, the stakeholders to be engaged might include those whose health is in question and/or a variety of actors who are responsible for or will sustain costs or benefits from efforts to improve health,

Disclosure: The authors have nothing to disclose.
[a] Duke Division of Community Health, Department of Family Medicine and Community Health, Duke Council on Race and Ethnicity, Duke University, DUMC 104652, Durham, NC 27710, USA;
[b] Duke Department of Family Medicine and Community Health, Duke University, DUMC 3886, 2100 Erwin Road, Durham, NC 27710, USA
* Corresponding author.
E-mail address: Mina.silberberg@duke.edu
twitter: @vivimbmd (V.M.-B.)

Prim Care Clin Office Pract 46 (2019) 587–594
https://doi.org/10.1016/j.pop.2019.07.014
0095-4543/19/© 2019 Elsevier Inc. All rights reserved.

such as providers, researchers, public health professionals, and policy makers. For the purposes of this article, the term stakeholder engagement is deemed to be inclusive of individuals, communities, and entities who in some way have a stake in the health issue in question.

One particular form of stakeholder engagement is engagement of the community whose health will be directly affected, often referred to as community engagement.[a] The US Centers for Disease Control and Prevention (CDC) defines community engagement as "the process of working collaboratively with and through groups of people affiliated by geographic proximity, special interest, or similar situations to address issues affecting the well-being of those people."[3]

Stakeholder-engaged research as a specific form of stakeholder-engaged population health improvement is increasingly promoted by funders such as the National Institutes of Health, the Patient Center Outcomes Research Institute, and the Robert Wood Johnson Foundation. Wallerstein and Duran[4] conceptualized a continuum of participatory or engaged research. On one end of the continuum is Kurt Lewin's action-research approach, which gives primacy to the benefits of engaged research for practical problem solving. Which stakeholders are engaged in this kind of study depends on the type of problem to be solved and the knowledge, relationships, and other resources necessary to effectively design, perform, and disseminate the research in a way that is likely to lead to action. On the other end of the continuum is research that adapts the pedagogical teachings of Paolo Freire to the research endeavor, encouraging groups that are marginalized by society to use action and reflection to develop their own understanding of and act on the conditions oppressing them. This kind of research puts a primacy on sharing power with the stakeholders who are most often thought of as the community. Community-based participatory research (CBPR), which involves affected communities as equal partners in all stages, lies at this end of the continuum.

A growing literature provides evidence for the benefits of stakeholder engagement for population health improvement.[3–8] This literature indicates that engagement:

- Increases the relevance of research questions and interventions
- Provides insight into health as part of a larger context
- Takes into account the needs, assets, and concerns of affected communities
- Encourages development of interventions that are tailored to the local context, nonduplicative, and sustainable
- Promotes relationships of trust and improves communication between researchers and practitioners
- Enlists new resources and allies
- Enhances research quality through stakeholder assistance with recruitment, the wording of research instruments, insights into the interpretation of results, and other support
- Strengthens community power
- Promotes immediate benefit to stakeholders in the form of compensation for their time, sharing of knowledge, and demystification of research and intervention processes

---

[a] The term community engagement can also be used to refer to stakeholder engagement more generally. As noted in the CDC's *Principles of Community Engagement*, the word community is sometimes used to refer to people who are affected by the health issues being addressed or in a more general way, for example, by referring to stakeholders such as academics, public health professionals, and policy makers as communities. Both uses have advantages. This article defines community engagement as engagement of the communities whose health is at stake and distinguishes this from stakeholder engagement more generally.

- Enhances dissemination of research findings, successful interventions, lessons learned
- Increases the likelihood that research results will be used
- Develops sustained collaborations that build capacity to address more challenging issues over time

In a systematic review, Cyril and colleagues[9] found that community-engaged health studies and interventions can lead to improvements in health behaviors, public health planning, health service access, health literacy, and the reduction of health inequalities when performed with effective community consultation and participation, including authentic power sharing, bidirectional learning, assets and needs assessment, and incorporation of the opinions of affected communities into protocols. The potential benefits of community engagement for population health initiatives in the primary care field specifically are underscored by the fact that health and illness occur in the community, with only an estimated 25% of people who experience injuries and symptoms of illness presenting to a physician's office (and only 1 in 800 being hospitalized in academic centers).[10] Understanding the experience of those not presenting to clinical care during early symptoms of diseases can lead to better interventions to improve health.

THE PRINCIPLES OF ENGAGEMENT

Several different individuals and entities have developed principles to support stakeholder engagement. For example, the CDC has identified 9 principles of community engagement.[3] Israel and colleagues[11] identified 9 principles for CBPR, and Minkler and Wallerstein[12] added 2 more, for a total of 11. Some institutions are developing their own principles. For example, Duke Health has created 6 principles for its faculty and staff to follow when they engage with the community.[13] There are also principles associated with community-oriented primary care.[14] Some entities have developed models of health improvement that combine principles of community engagement with a focus on health equity. For example, the Multnomah County Health Department's Health Equity and Empowerment Lens is designed to lead to the development of racially equitable policies and programs through transformative processes that include community engagement and leadership by people of color.[15]

There is important variation in the principles that different practitioners bring to engagement. To a large extent, this variation corresponds to the differences in the philosophy and purpose of engagement represented in the continuum from action research to CBPR. However, there are also some common elements among the different sets of principles. These elements can be summarized as power sharing, respect, humility, colearning, commitment, and a goal of making change. Three examples of principles of community engagement are provided in **Boxes 1–3**.

EXAMPLES OF ENGAGEMENT

The concept of stakeholder engagement can seem abstract or intimidating. This article offers 3 examples of primary care providers engaging with other stakeholders to improve population health through synergistic collaboration. As these examples show, primary care engagement with other stakeholders can take a variety of forms, and can be initiated/led by primary care providers or their partners.

University of Illinois Health Pilsen Food Pantry

Evelyn Figueroa, a family physician at the University of Illinois (UI) in Chicago started the Pilsen Food Pantry at her medical clinic after learning about a similar undertaking

> **Box 1**
> **Centers for Disease Control and Prevention, principles of community engagement, 2011**
>
> 1. Be clear about the purposes or goals of the engagement effort and the populations and/or communities you want to engage.
>
> 2. Become knowledgeable about the community's culture, economic conditions, social networks, political and power structures, norms and values, demographic trends, history, and experience with efforts by outside groups to engage it in various programs. Learn about the community's perceptions of those initiating the engagement activities.
>
> 3. Go to the community, establish relationships, build trust, work with the formal and informal leadership, and seek commitment from community organizations and leaders to create processes for mobilizing the community.
>
> 4. Remember and accept that collective self-determination is the responsibility and right of all people in a community. No external entity should assume it can bestow on a community the power to act in its own self-interest.
>
> 5. Partnering with the community is necessary to create change and improve health.
>
> 6. All aspects of community engagement must recognize and respect the diversity of the community. Awareness of the various cultures of a community and other factors affecting diversity must be paramount in planning, designing, and implementing approaches to engaging a community.
>
> 7. Community engagement can only be sustained by identifying and mobilizing community assets and strengths and by developing the community's capacity and resources to make decisions and take action.
>
> 8. Organizations that wish to engage a community as well as individuals seeking to effect change must be prepared to release control of actions or interventions to the community and be flexible enough to meet its changing needs.
>
> 9. Community collaboration requires long-term commitment by the engaging organization and its partners.
>
> *From* CTSA Community Engagement Key Function Committee Task Force on the Principles of Community Engagement, ed Principles of Community Engagement, 2nd edition. Bethesda, MD: National Institutes of Health; 2011. Available at: https://www.atsdr.cdc.gov/communityengagement/pdf/PCE_Report_508_FINAL.pdf

at the University of California at San Diego.[16,17] To create the pantry, she partnered with the UI Health Pilsen Lower West Family Health Center, Trader Joe's, Imperfect Produce, the Greater Chicago Food Depository, and others. Launched in January of 2018, the pantry is open for 4 hours 5 days a week, and is staffed primarily by volunteers, who include medical students, residents, members of the university's volunteer services, and individuals from the community; in August of 2019, a part-time manager was hired, the pantry's first employee. Food is provided to the pantry from grocery rescues, food drives, and Greater Chicago, or is bought by the pantry at low cost. All food is free to pantry visitors. In 2018, the pantry distributed more than 90,900 kg (200,000 pounds) of food to more than 6000 individuals. The food pantry also supplies feminine hygiene products through partnership with the Chicago Period Project, and a women's, infants, and children's (WIC) office is colocated with the pantry to help connect women to WIC and the Supplemental Nutrition Assistance Program. Medical students conduct cooking classes quarterly.

The Boston Safe Shops Project

In the early 2000s, the Boston Public Health Commission (BPHC) determined from citizen complaints, inspections, and community advocates that the pollution impact for

---

Box 2
Guiding principles of community-oriented primary care

1. Local health, not panel of patients. Orient the care and analysis of health outcomes to the health and health care of a defined population or community. Focus on all people within a defined community rather than just those who are actively coming to the clinic or health system as patients.

2. Comprehensive care based on identified health needs at the population level. Identify health problems by population-level (rather than only clinic-level) metrics and consider the perspective of community members. Including health promotion, disease prevention, and treatment of disease.

3. Prioritize health equity. Priority health concerns should be determined jointly by health care professionals and community members. Promote equity in health: design care that is accessible, appropriate, affordable, and relevant.

4. Practice with science. Interdisciplinary and multiprofessional practice teams, using evidence to cover all stages of the health-illness continuum.

5. Service integration around users. Integrate services around users, work with the community and not just in the community. Engage in dialogue and mutual respect, recognize autonomy and agency, and collaborate continuously with community organizations to increase the likelihood that interventions will be sustainable and effective.

Data from Marcus T. COPC – a practical guide. Pretoria, South Africa: Department of Family Medicine, University of Pretoria; 2018.

Box 3
Principles of community-based participatory research

1. Recognizes community as a unit of identity.

2. Builds on strengths and resources within the community.

3. Facilitates a collaborative, equitable partnership in all phases of research, involving an empowering and power-sharing process that attends to social inequalities.

4. Fosters colearning and capacity building among all partners.

5. Integrates and achieves a balance between knowledge generation and intervention for the mutual benefit of all partners.

6. Focuses on the local relevance of public health problems and on ecological perspectives that attend to the multiple determinants of health.

7. Involves systems development using a cyclical and iterative process.

8. Disseminates results to all partners and involves them in the wider dissemination of results.

9. Involves a long-term process and commitment to sustainability.

10. Openly addresses issues of race, ethnicity, racism, and social class, and embodies cultural humility.

11. Works to ensure research rigor and validity but also seeks to "broaden the bandwidth of validity" with respect to research relevance.

Data from Israel BA, Schulz AJ, Parker EA, et al. Review of community-based research: assessing partnership approaches to improve public health. Annu. Rev. Public Health. 1998;19(1):173-202; and Minkler M, Wallerstein N. Community-based participatory research for health: from process to outcomes. 2nd ed. San Francisco: Jossey-Bass; 2008.

> **Box 4**
> **Tools for further learning on stakeholder engagement**
>
> 1. Clinical and Translational Science Awards Community Engagement Key Function Committee Task Force on the Principles of Community Engagement. *Principles of Community Engagement, second edition.* Bethesda, MD: National Institutes of Health, 2011 (#11–7782). Also available at: https://www.atsdr.cdc.gov/communityengagement/pdf/PCE_Report_508_FINAL.pdf
>
> 2. Wallerstein, Nina, Bonnie Duran, John G. Oetzel, and Meredith Minkler, eds. *Community-Based Participatory Research for Health: Advancing Social and Health Equity, third edition.* San Francisco: John Wiley and Sons, 2018.
>
> 3. Israel, Barbara A., Eugenia Eng, Amy J. Schulz, and Edith J. Parker. *Methods for Community-Based Participatory Research for Health, second edition.* San Francisco: John Wiley and Sons, 2013.
>
> 4. The Practical Playbook, at https://www.practicalplaybook.org
>
> 5. Community Tool Box, at https://ctb.ku.edu/en
>
> 6. Community-Campus Partnerships for Health, at https://www.ccphealth.org/
>
> 7. Health Research & Educational Trust. *Hospital-based Strategies for Creating a Culture of Health.* Chicago, IL: Health Research & Educational Trust, 2014 (October).
>
> 8. Institute of Medicine. *Primary Care and Public Health: Exploring Integration to Improve Population Health. A report of the Committee on Integrating Primary Care and Public Health; Board on Population Health and Public Health Practice; Institute of Medicine.* Washington (DC): National Academies Press (United States), 2012 (March).
>
> 9. Journal: *Progress in Community Health Partnerships: Research, Education, and Action.*
>
> 10. *Partnering to Catalyze Comprehensive Community Wellness: An Actionable Framework for Health Care and Public Health Collaboration.* Available at https://hcttf.org/wp-content/uploads/2018/06/Comprehensive-Community-Wellness-Report.pdf.
>
> 11. The Everyone Project AAFP Toolkit https://www.aafp.org/patient-care/social-determinants-of-health/everyone-project/eop-tools/community-collaboration.html.

neighbors of small automotive shops, and chemical exposure and injuries among shop employees, were an important concern.[18–20] BPHC developed a multisectoral partnership that included an occupational health physician from Uphams' Corner Community Health Center. The Safe Shops Project offers small automotive stores the opportunity to learn how to protect their workers, save money, and reduce their impact on the neighborhood environment. Initially, shops were given the opportunity to host a public health van for a day to provide screenings and health education to workers, their families, customers, and neighbors, and link them to health care if needed; although valuable, that program was eventually discontinued because of high operation costs and decreased need resulting from Massachusetts's health insurance mandate and efforts to achieve full coverage in the state. BPHC has reached out to community health centers across the city to inform physicians of the program and the resources it provides to small businesses. In 2007, the Safe Shops Project published results indicating improvements in shop conditions, personnel knowledge, and practices. The Safe Shops Program expanded to include nail salons in 2007 and hair salons in 2017.

Whitman-Walker: A Study in Medical-Legal Partnership and Policy Change

Whitman-Walker Health (Washington, DC) is a health center that specializes in care for the Lesbian, Gay, Bisexual, Transgender, and Questioning or Queer community.[21–23]

It is also one of the hundreds of clinical sites that has embraced medical-legal partnership. At Whitman-Walker, the oldest medical-legal partnership in the nation, on-site legal services help patients address issues related to health insurance, work disputes, discrimination, public benefits, immigration, powers of attorney and wills, elder issues, identity documents for transgender clients, and more. In addition to addressing the needs of individual patients, the medical-legal partnership works to systemically reform policies that negatively affect their patients. One example stemmed from providers and pharmacists at Whitman-Walker working to ensure that people who are exposed to human immunodeficiency virus (HIV) take postexposure prophylaxis (PEP) medication within 72 hours of the exposure to keep them HIV negative. Whitman-Walker found that 2 of the health plans used by their patients only provided PEP as a mail-order drug, meaning it would arrive long after that critical exposure window had closed. Whitman-Walker pharmacists and insurance navigators worked with the operations and legal teams to contact the health plan and request that PEP prescriptions be filled immediately, and not through mail order. Within a week, both plans had changed their policies, leading to more efficient and timely access to PEP.

CONTINUING TO LEARN ABOUT ENGAGEMENT

This article provides a brief introduction to stakeholder engagement, but there is an ever-widening pool of resources available to help clinicians who wish to enhance their skills in this area. Some of those tools are identified in **Box 4**.

REFERENCES

1. Hanson P. Citizen involvement in community health promotion: a role application of CDC's PATCH model. Int Q Community Health Educ 1988;9(3):177–86.
2. Institute of Medicine. The future of public health. Washington, DC: National Academy Press; 1988.
3. CTSA Community Engagement Key Function Committee Task Force on the Principles of Community Engagement. Principles of Community Engagement, 2nd edition. Bethesda (MD): National Institutes of Health; 2011. #11-7782.
4. Wallerstein N, Duran B. The theoretical, historical, and practice roots of CBPR. In: Wallerstein N, Duran B, Oetzel J, et al, editors. Community-based participatory research for health: advancing social and health equity. 3rd edition. San Francisco (CA): Jossey Bass; 2017. p. 17–29.
5. Shore N. Re-conceptualizing the Belmont Report: a community-based participatory research perspective. J Community Pract 2006;14(4):5–26.
6. Wallerstein N. Empowerment to reduce health disparities. Scand J Public Health 2002;30:72–7.
7. Viswanathan M, Ammerman A, Eng E, et al. Community-based participatory research: assessing the evidence. Rockville (MD): AHRQ; 2004.
8. Staley K. Exploring impact: public involvement in NHS, public health and social care research. Eastleigh (England): INVOLVE; 2009.
9. Cyril S, Smith B, Possamai-Inesedy A, et al. Exploring the role of community engagement in improving the health of disadvantaged populations: a systematic review. Glob Health Action 2015;8:29842.
10. Green L, Fryer G, Yawn B, et al. The ecology of medical care revisited. N Engl J Med 2001;344(26):2021–5.
11. Israel BA, Schulz AJ, Parker EA, et al. Review of community-based research: assessing partnership approaches to improve public health. Annu Rev Public Health 1998;19(1):173–202.

12. Minkler M, Wallerstein N. Community-based participatory research for health: from process to outcomes. 2nd edition. San Francisco (CA): Jossey-Bass; 2008.

13. Principles of community engagement. Available at: https://communityrelations.duhs.duke.edu/principles-community-engagement. Accessed December 20, 2018.

14. Marcus T. COPC – a practical guide. Pretoria (South Africa): Department of Family Medicine, University of Pretoria; 2018.

15. Equity and empowerment lens logic model. 2014. Available at: https://multco.us/file/31825/download. Accessed December 22, 2018.

16. UI Health Pilsen Food Pantry - Chicago, IL. Available at: https://www.figueroawufamilyfoundation.com/food-pantry/. Accessed December 27, 2018.

17. Email Communication between Mina Silberberg and Evelyn Figueroa. December 27-28, 2018.

18. Shoemaker PA, Skogstrom T, Shea J, et al. The Boston safe shops project–preliminary findings of a case study in applying the 10 essential services of public health to building environmental health capacity. J Environ Health 2007;70(1):22–8.

19. BPHC. Safe shops. Available at: http://www.bphc.org/whatwedo/healthy-homes-environment/safe-shops/Pages/Safe-Shops.aspx. Accessed April 29, 2019.

20. Email Communication between Mina Silberberg and Hibo Dahir. February 4, 2019.

21. Marple K, Dexter E. Eliminating hurdles to live-saving medication. A Report of the National Center for Medical-Legal Partnership; 2018.

22. Whitman-Walker Health. Available at: https://www.whitman-walker.org/. Accessed December 26, 2018.

23. Email Communication between Mina Silberberg and Naseema Shafi. January 9, 2019.

Models of Population Health

Lisa P. Shock, DrPH(c), MHS, PA-C[a,b,c,*]

KEYWORDS

- Population health • Models of population health • Value-based care

KEY POINTS

- This article discusses innovative models of population health, reviewing the change from fee for service to fee for value.
- It is critical to place emphasis on population health innovation as well as reformed clinical delivery, stressing quality of care.
- Successful models of population health management programs use community engagement tools and address social determinants of health.

INTRODUCTION

Since the development of the triple aim framework by the Institute for Health Improvement in Cambridge, Massachusetts, innovative health systems and community programs have begun to address population health.[1] Development of varying models of population health has been prolific since the original definition in 2003 by Kindig and Stoddart[2] describing population health as "the health outcomes of a group of individuals, including the distribution of such outcomes within the group." This original definition did not define population health in terms of clinical populations, drawing attention away from the critical role that nonclinical factors, such as education and economic development, play in producing health.[3] For this reason, Kindig[3] modified his own definition in 2015, encouraging the term population health management or,

Disclosure: The author's title at Evolent Health is Vice President, Clinical Strategy & Operations, Value Based Care. The author oversees and manages clinical teams delivering value-based clinical programs in partnership with health systems across the nation. Her academic involvement as a consulting faculty member at Duke as well as her pursuit of a DrPH degree at UNC are not job requirements, nor have they been recommended by her employer for job advancement. Evolent Health does not financially support her education. All opinions stated within this work are the author's own and this work is an independent work product, done outside of her regular job responsibilities

[a] Evolent Health, Clinical Strategy & Operations, Value Based Care, Raleigh, NC, USA; [b] Duke University Medical Center, Geriatrics Education Center, Durham, NC, USA; [c] Department of Health Policy & Management, University of North Carolina, Gillings School of Global Public Health, Chapel Hill, NC, USA
* 3128 Smoketree Court, Raleigh, NC 27604, USA.
E-mail address: lisa.shock@gmail.com

Prim Care Clin Office Pract 46 (2019) 595–602
https://doi.org/10.1016/j.pop.2019.07.011
0095-4543/19/© 2019 Elsevier Inc. All rights reserved.

perhaps even better, population medicine to better reflect measurements of health outcomes rather than a defined geographic subpopulation.

True population health management cannot be realized by health care systems acting alone, nor by solely delivering high-quality care at lower costs. Successful models of population health must not myopically focus on care delivery but must also seek to engage partners across their communities to address community culture as well as the broader social determinants of health (SDOH). Modern models of population health must incorporate both innovation as well as reform in the clinical delivery process. Use of team-based care, targeted population interventions, and creativity in redesigned incentives are core competencies necessary to effectively change the way health care is delivered across populations.

POPULATION HEALTH MODELS AS DRIVERS FOR CLINICAL DELIVERY REFORM: TEAM-BASED CARE

In value, accountable care, and shared savings, the overarching goal is to increase delivery of quality health care at an affordable, sustainable cost. Examples may include appropriate triage of nonemergent patients away from the emergency department and instead back to a primary care provider with extended office hours, or use of care coordination in chronically ill populations, which may also be condition focused with special programs around heart failure or diabetes. Changing incentives through insurance redesign can allow health systems and provider groups to be rewarded for prevention with care coordination incentives that are foreign to the fee-for-service mindset.

Interdisciplinary teams of new health care workers, including population health managers and care coordinators, have emerged. Clinical delivery within models of population health often use an interdisciplinary approach with physician assistants (PAs) and nurse practitioners (NPs), social workers, and community health workers addressing both physical health as well as social determinants. The focus in these new delivery models is not on what is done to patients, but true quality and outcomes measurement. Incentives reward performance on quality measures and care coordination through patient transitions such as hospitalizations or surgery.

Nationwide, hospitals and health systems are also expanding health care delivery teams by using more PAs and NPs and there is a much greater emphasis on team-based, interdisciplinary care. Increasing capacity of the health system to meet the growing numbers of patients seeking care is critical and necessary. In the team-based care model, all care team members participate in delivery of health services by working at the top of their licensure and skill set. For example, PAs and NPs can be empaneled, offering primary care delivery services; nurses can conduct complex care management and patient education programs; front desk staff can call patients who need evidence-based care quality gaps to be closed; medical assistants can provide medication review, goal setting, patient education, and electronic health record scribing; and pharmacists can support complex medication reconciliation and comprehensive medication management programs.[4] Implementing interdisciplinary care teams is a critical element of transforming a practice into a patient-centered medical home. Leveraging the entire care team, including families and community partners, allows the primary care medical home to design efficient and important outreach processes more effectively to support patient health goals.

Leveraging a team approach to care allows the physician and other members of the team to focus on diagnosis and treatment and allows others to relieve some of the administrative burden. There is mounting evidence that nonphysician members of a care team more effectively provide many care coordination activities. A single primary care provider would need greater than 18 h/d to address and provide all of the evidence-based preventive and chronic illness care required for an average panel of patients.[5] Other evidence shows that most providers spend 13% of their days on care coordination activities and only 50% of their time on activities using their medical knowledge.[6]

Challenges to building effective infrastructure and amassing appropriate resources are felt more acutely by smaller, more rural providers. Value-based accountable care programs are initiated more quickly in larger physician groups and hospital systems for these reasons. Newer federal incentives such as the Practice Transformation Network initiative encourage and incentivize resource allocation to these providers.[7] In 2015, The Centers for Medicare & Medicaid Services (CMS) awarded $685 million to 39 national and regional collaborative health care transformation networks and supporting organizations to provide technical assistance, which will enable more than 140,000 clinicians and their practices with resources designed to support value-based practice transformation.

POPULATION HEALTH MODELS: TARGETED POPULATIONS

Redesigned models of population health include stratification of populations by age, disease, plan coverage/benefits, and geography. An example of a targeted population based on age and health coverage is Medicare. Medicare population growth is significant and leaves many older patients facing access issues. Between 2012 and 2050, the United States will experience considerable growth in its older population. By 2050, one-fifth of the total US population will be elderly (that is, 65 years of age or older), up from 12% in 2000 and 8% in 1950.[8] The baby boomers are largely responsible for this increase in the older population, because they began turning 65 years old in 2011.

The need to control excess health care spending in this population led to innovative payment models under the Centers for Medicare & Medicaid Services (CMS), the most common of which is the genesis of accountable care organizations (ACOs). Health reform efforts focused on value-based care have led to a significant proliferation of ACOs nationwide over the last several years. Since the passage of the Affordable Care Act, ACOs are now an established new payment model under Medicare.[9] ACOs will allow physicians, hospitals, and other clinicians together with community health care organizations to work more effectively together to both improve quality and slow spending growth for a defined population of Medicare beneficiaries.[9] ACOs are specifically defined as health care entities that make efforts to reduce fee-for-service Medicare spending through care and cost improvement efforts.[10] ACOs may be composed of any combination of hospitals, health systems, and independent physician associations under an ACO governance structure delivering coordinated care. Participation in Medicare Shared Savings Programs with CMS has been associated with significant reductions in postacute spending without "ostensible deterioration in quality of care."[11] Spending reductions remained consistent with clinicians working within hospitals and skilled nursing facilities to influence care for ACO attributed patients.[11]

CORE COMPETENCIES OF CULTURE AND IDENTIFICATION OF SOCIAL DETERMINANTS OF HEALTH

Addressing culture when designing health interventions and new models of population health is largely accepted as important and often critical to successful patient outcomes. For example, when considering the vulnerable elderly, there is a need to understand their culture through a method similar to Asad and Kay's[12] work, which recommends that efforts "not only account for local variation, but also provide a concrete framework for those interested in implementing health interventions across diverse geographic, ethno-racial, and political settings."[12] Asad and Kay[12] maintain that in order to successfully affect health outcomes, health interventions must be implemented in a way that is sensitive to that population's health-seeking behavior.

For example, the elderly population has a higher use of health resources. By encouraging clinician and team awareness of cultural practice, health interventions can be influenced, and individual patient outcomes improved for this population. As Asad and Kay[12] maintain, "Not only must groups of individuals share cultural knowledge, but through their interactions with one another, they must also select the knowledge they need and what they do with it. While individuals' choices are generally enabled or constrained by structural forces, individuals also have the potential to facilitate structural and cultural changes."[6]

Structural change related to culture in the US health care system is also evident in new government standards that are being incorporated into new models of population health. The National Standards for Culturally and Linguistically Appropriate Services (CLAS) in Health and Health Care are intended to improve health care quality and advance health equity by establishing a framework for organizations to serve the nation's increasingly diverse communities.[7] Training health care teams on these standards through education, governance, and leadership while promoting culturally and linguistically appropriate policies and practices on an ongoing basis is another avenue toward improving cultural awareness for diverse populations. In addition to using continuing education efforts,[13] and understanding cross-cultural efforts,[14] adopting national efforts driven by the CLAS framework will be necessary to engage an informed clinical workforce to create new models of care.

Innovative models of population health must often address geographic nuances within health and wellness initiatives. Risky health behaviors in rural communities suggest a cultural component of rural health that is described by Hartley[15] as a "rural culture determinant." This model presents an illustrative example of integrated rural health that draws influences from the traditionally defined social determinant components of people, place, and equitable opportunity,[16] as well as the added impacts of patient activation, health literacy, community engagement, risk stratification, and provider preparedness.

Existing frameworks, such as THRIVE the (Tool for Health and Resilience in Vulnerable Environments[16]) address SDOH through community-informed, measurable, and actionable resilience assessments. THRIVE implementation and training efforts occurred across 12 public health institutes and communities across the United States since 2012 and examined a model of health defined by structural drivers (power, money, and resource allocation) as well as community-level daily living conditions (education, employment, food, housing). Other efforts to model SDOH categorize determinants into biology, environment, lifestyle, and health care organization.[17] Many current models of population health account for these social factors.

Newer approaches expand and cite the influences of individual patient behaviors and activation and also include the significant impacts of family and culture on substance abuse, smoking habits, sexual heath, physical activity, and nutrition on the greater community. Added considerations within the domain of the physical environment include the example influences of environment (air, water, pollution) as well as physical (safety, overcrowding) and chemical (lead paint exposure, pollutants) determinants. Models of population health that are successful in both cost savings and improved quality of health care delivery address these important influences.

Economics of both individual and community are addressed within the domain of equitable opportunity, and access to care is a critical factor in most models of population health. Availability and exposure to adequate education and occupation directly affect social factors, including socioeconomic status and the concept of applied social capital to overall community health. It is important not only to consider the generalized availability of health services but also to incorporate the need for the greater medical community to address issues of access to care. Emphasis in planning on regional, local, and state efforts to examine usage patterns and target community interventions and strategies based on risk is important to implementation model success. In addition, the component of provider preparedness and awareness of SDOH is critical to local success and must be addressed both in the organic community as well as within formalized interprofessional education and training across the health delivery system.

Changing access to care through improved delivery models by improving the social perception of vulnerable populations and increasing the cultural awareness and cultural competence of the health care delivery team is an ambitious goal. Displacing the tradition and values of rationalization through improved interdisciplinary training and concrete cultural awareness efforts will mitigate the rationalization of these populations. Through national, local, and individual efforts, clinicians can influence and improve cultural awareness and adjust their systemic processes to better address gaps in knowledge, literacy, and access to care. With continued attention to culture and diversity, clinicians will improve their understanding of diversity and, ultimately, improve overall delivery of health care services and achieve improved health across populations.

POPULATION HEALTH MANAGEMENT: CREATIVITY IN REDESIGNED INCENTIVES

To implement truly innovative models of population health, there is a need for better measurement and realistic targets as part of practice redesign in the name of quality care delivery, with the goal of overall health outcomes improvement. Payment reform is a necessary component of an accurate measure of the associations between practice transformation and health outcomes for both patients and society.[18]

In 2008, Berwick and colleagues[19] proposed that the US health care system adopt a triple aim: to improve health care, to improve population health, and to reduce per capita health care costs. The formulation of the triple aim responds to 3 main problems facing the US health care system: high cost, low quality, and poor health status.[20] Addressing the triple aim is the latest and most ambitious effort toward systemic payment reform, which progressed from cost containment in the 1970s, to cost containment while/by improving quality in the 1980s and 1990s, to cost containment while/by improving quality and population health most recently.[20] From CMS's perspective, the triple aim is vital to Medicare, and new value-based payment systems, including the ACO, have been deployed to achieve it.

ACOs and hospitals are currently investing in improving population health, by which they mean they are addressing the health of the population of patients attributed by Medicare, Medicaid, or private health insurers to their organizations.[21] However, population health can and should also encompass "the health of the entire population in a geographic area."[21]

In the past, US hospitals and physicians have focused primarily on an encounter-based, fee-for-service payment system, which pays for services provided to patients during a visit or hospitalization.[21] At present, ACOs are also paid on a fee-for-service basis, but they are, in addition, given substantial financial incentives by payers to try to contain the overall costs of patients' care and to improve the quality of care delivery, particularly for patients with chronic illnesses, such as diabetes.[21] These added financial benefits give hospitals and physicians that participate in these value-based ACO contracts an incentive to identify all of their attributed patients who should be receiving care and encourages them to provide care not only during face-to-face visits but also via phone, e-mail, and contact with nurse care managers specially trained to assist patients with chronic illnesses.[21] This shift in incentives drives ACOs to work proactively and systematically toward improving their patients' health outcomes, and it is this framework that engenders continued enthusiasm for models of population health among the ACO leadership.[22]

Future models of population health must support ACOs and hospitals investing in programs affecting the socioeconomic determinants of health to improve the health of the population in their geographic area. Policy efforts at the state, local, and national levels will influence the availability of resources and access to funding to assist the addressing of population SDOH. Community engagement and advocacy efforts will be necessary to build healthier communities and enact social change.

Online resources, such as the community tool box, offer educational modules and resources to promote community development[23] and assist health system leaders in defining strategic interventions. Effective future policy interventions must also address geographic variation and be based on defined differences faced by rural communities. When arguing for a "progressive rhetoric for rural America, " Ricketts noted that urban-rural comparisons are "plagued by the problem of aggregation of widely divergent nonmetropolitan populations" while there remain "regional patterns of rural disadvantage."[24]

Effective and future changes in models of population health must comprise high-quality care at the most affordable cost as well as efficient cooperation, innovation, and health promotion.[25] In order to stimulate value in the broadest sense, and implement new models of population health, 2 components of incentives must be addressed: a risk-adjusted global base payment with risk-sharing elements paid to a multidisciplinary provider group for the provision of the full continuum of care to a designated, attributed population,[25] and a lower-powered variable payment that explicitly rewards aspects of value that can be adequately measured, such as (1) high-quality care, (2) cost-conscious behavior, (3) well-coordinated care, (4) cost-effective innovation, and (5) cost-effective prevention.[25]

Present-day hospitals and health systems are limited in their incentives, capabilities, and authority to take primary responsibility for the health of their attributed populations spanning their geographic areas. ACOs and health systems could be important partners in population health organization coalitions assuming responsibility for the health of their geographic populations. These coalitions and systemic changes will not be easy to create or to fund; the belief that they could exist may seem excessively optimistic.[26] However, it is critical to remain optimistic if reform efforts are to create new models of population health delivery and catalyze new health policy for the future.

REFERENCES

1. Institute for Healthcare Improvement: IHI Home Page. Available at: http://www.ihi.org/Pages/default.aspx. Accessed December 10, 2018.
2. Kindig D, Stoddart G. What is population health? Am J Public Health 2003;93(3): 380–3. Available at: http://www.ncbi.nlm.nih.gov/pubmed/12604476. Accessed December 10, 2018.

3. Kindig DA. What are we talking about when we talk about population health?. Available at: https://www.healthaffairs.org/do/10.1377/hblog20150406.046151/full/. Accessed December 10, 2018.
4. Safety Net Medical Home Staff. Safety net medical home initiative. Available at: http://www.safetynetmedicalhome.org/sites/default/files/Implementation-Guide-Supplement-Team-Based-Care.pdf. Accessed December 10, 2018.
5. Yarnall KS, Ostbye T, Krause KM, et al. Family physicians as team leaders: "time" to share the care. Prev Chronic Dis 2009;6(2):59.
6. Bodenheimer T, Laing BY. The teamlet model of primary care. Ann Fam Med 2007,5(5):457–61.
7. CMS Staff. Transforming clinical practice initiative. CMS.gov. Available at: https://innovation.cms.gov/initiatives/Transforming-Clinical-Practices/. Accessed December 10, 2018.
8. CBO Staff. Rising demand for long term services and supports for elderly people. Available at: https://www.cbo.gov/publication/44363. Accessed December 10, 2018.
9. Fisher ES, Shortell SM. Accountable care organizations. JAMA 2010;304(15):1715.
10. Pham HH, Cohen M, Conway PH, et al. The pioneer accountable care organization model. JAMA 2014;312(16):1635.
11. McWilliams JM, Gilstrap LG, Stevenson DG, et al. Changes in postacute care in the medicare shared savings program. JAMA Intern Med 2017;177(4):518–26.
12. Asad AL, Kay T. Toward a multidimensional understanding of culture for health interventions. Soc Sci Med 2015;144:79–87.
13. Salman A, McCabe D, Easter T, et al. Cultural competence among staff nurses who participated in a family-centered geriatric care program. J Nurses Staff Dev 2007;23(3):103–11.
14. Surbone A, Kagawa-Singer M, Terret C, et al. The illness trajectory of elderly cancer patients across cultures: SIOG position paper. Ann Oncol 2006;18(4):633–8.
15. Hartley D. Rural health disparities, population health, and rural culture. Am J Public Health 2004;94(10):1675–8.
16. THRIVE: tool for health & resilience in vulnerable environments | prevention institute. Available at: https://www.preventioninstitute.org/tools/thrive-tool-health-resilience-vulnerable-environments. Accessed December 22, 2018.
17. Young TK. Population health: concepts and methods. New York: Oxford University Press; 2004.
18. Huerta TR, Hefner JL, McAlearney AS. Payment models to support population health management. Adv Health Care Manag 2014;16:177–83. Available at: http://www.ncbi.nlm.nih.gov/pubmed/25626206. Accessed December 22, 2018.
19. Berwick DM, Nolan TW, Whittington J. The triple aim: care, health, and cost. Health Aff 2008;27(3):759–69.
20. Tanenbaum SJ. Can payment reform be social reform? The lure and liabilities of the "Triple Aim." J Health Polit Policy Law 2017;42(1):53–71.
21. Noble DJ, Greenhalgh T, Casalino LP. Improving population health one person at a time? Accountable care organisations: perceptions of population health—a qualitative interview study. BMJ Open 2014;4(4):e004665.
22. Crosson FJ. The accountable care organization: whatever its growing pains, the concept is too vitally important to fail. Health Aff 2011;30(7):1250–5.
23. The community tool box. Available at: https://ctb.ku.edu/en/build-your-toolbox. Accessed December 24, 2018.

24. Ricketts TC. Arguing for rural health in medicare: a progressive rhetoric for rural America. J Rural Heal 2004;20(1):43–51.
25. Cattel D, Eijkenaar F, Schut FT. Value-based provider payment: towards a theoretically preferred design. Heal Econ Policy Law 2018;1–19. https://doi.org/10.1017/S1744133118000397.
26. Casalino LP, Erb N, Joshi MS, et al. Accountable care organizations and population health organizations. J Health Polit Policy Law 2015;40(4):821–37.

Health Care Value

Relationships Between Population Health, Patient Experience, and Costs of Care

Reshma Gupta, MD, MSHPM[a,b,*]

KEYWORDS

- Health-care value • Quality of care for populations • Patient experience
- Affordability • Prices

KEY POINTS

- Health care delivery has become fragmented, varied, and expensive. National health care gross domestic product and out-of-pocket expenses are increasing exponentially without improved quality outcomes compared with similar nations.
  - Health care value captures the quality of health for populations, patient experiences, and the expenses of care, and each component is vital to achieve high-value care delivery.
  - Different stakeholders in the health care system view the meaning of quality care for populations, experience, and costs differently.
  - High-quality care is best delivered based on understanding the needs of a practice's patient population and keeping them healthy in the outpatient setting, which in return can reduce costs and improve patient experience.
  - Having parallel efforts to both reduce total costs of care and improve patient affordability can help improve population health and patient experience goals.

Mrs P is a grandmother of 3 children and is their primary caregiver. Her daughter works two different jobs to pay the bills and is rarely at home. Mrs P is a relatively healthy 84-year-old who enjoys spending time at home with the children and generally believes in living a "simple life" at her age. Over the last day she developed an uncomplicated diarrhea with no fever, bleeding, travel, or other significant medical conditions and went to her local emergency department for evaluation. A clinician ordered a computed tomographic (CT) scan of her abdomen, which found no source of infection. The patient was treated with fluids, antinausea medication,

[a] UCLA Health, 10945 Le Conte Avenue, Suite 1401, Los Angeles, CA 90095, USA; [b] Division of General Internal Medicine and Health Services Research, David Geffen School of Medicine, University of California Los Angeles, Los Angeles, CA, USA
* 10945 Le Conte Ave, Suite 1401, Los Angeles, CA 90095.
E-mail address: R44gupta@ucla.edu

Prim Care Clin Office Pract 46 (2019) 603–622
https://doi.org/10.1016/j.pop.2019.07.005
0095-4543/19/© 2019 Elsevier Inc. All rights reserved.

primarycare.theclinics.com

and was sent home a few hours later. The final read of the CT scan happened to incidentally identify a nodule on their pancreas, which sent her down the road of multiple follow-up appointments with specialists, further imaging that did not help to decipher the nodule, and a biopsy. She and her daughter struggled to make the appointments, losing wages and paying extra for childcare to take Mrs P into the clinic. Mrs P underwent the biopsy, but it was complicated by significant bleeding that required blood transitions and a stay in the hospital overnight. The biopsy results reported that the tissue was normal without evidence of malignancy.

Mrs P trusts her doctors and care team and followed all recommendations. However, she and her daughter expressed that they never understood why the doctors order the scan in the emergency department or the biopsy, and she reported that no one had asked her goals of care before. Weeks later she received 3 bills in the mail from the medical center that she and her daughter could not afford. Mrs P reported feeling that she wished she had never come to the emergency department that day. (Patient Story obtained from Dr Gupta).

INTRODUCTION

Health care in the United States is fraught with complexity, fragmentation, inefficiency, unexplained variation, and waste. In order to navigate this complexity in ways that make care more affordable, safe, and convenient for patient populations, patients and their caregivers will need to understand how to deliver and receive high-value care. This will require understanding how health care value is defined, the relationship between population health and high-value care, and opportunities for improvement across different health care stakeholders.

Since the turn of the twenty-first century there has been a growing desire for increased accountability in health care to achieve the goals of high-value care or the triple aim for patient populations (ie, quality of health for populations, patient experience, and costs of health care).[1] Initially, 2 landmark papers from the Institute of Medicine, Crossing the Quality Chasm and To Err is Human, galvanized quality and safety improvement and later patient experience.[2,3] Increasingly, although, there has been growing scrutiny over the exorbitant spending to achieve these goals in caring for patient populations. Various stakeholders realize that the over $3 trillion annual gross domestic product (GDP) health care expenditures (17.2% of total GDP)—highest among Organization for Economic Cooperation and Development countries—and the increased cost shifting to patients and employers is not sustainable (**Fig. 1**).[4] This article focuses on understanding the relationship between population health, patient experience, and the costs of delivering health care. It also discusses nuanced approaches to achieving high-value care for patient populations from different stakeholder perspectives since all groups have a vital role in improving outcomes.

Defining Health Care Value

Health care value has broadly been defined as health care outcomes per unit of cost.[5] "Value" is an overarching term that captures the quality of health for populations, patient experience, and costs of care. Each component is vital to achieve high-value care delivery. For decades, health systems have focused on improving quality and experience for their patients; however, with rising costs. Now in some settings, expensive health systems are losing business to more affordable, higher-quality providers.

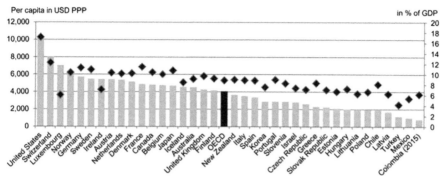

Fig. 1. Health spending per capita and as share of GDP, 2017. Bar graph represents health spending per capital. Diamonds represent share of GDP (%). Data for 2017 was estimated by the Secretariat for those countries that were not able to provide this information. PPP stands for Purchasing Power Parities and adjusts health expenditure for differences in price levels between countries. OECD (Organization for Economic Co-operation and Development) consists of 34 countries, including members characterized as emerging economies. (*From* OECD (2018), Mueller M, Morgan D. Focus on Spending on Health: Latest Trends, http://www.oecd.org/health/health-systems/Health-Spending-Latest-Trends-Brief.pdf; with permission.)

"VALUE" DOES NOT EQUATE TO "COSTS"

"Value," however, is often conflated into meaning costs alone. There are, however, numerous scenarios in which this conflation is inaccurate. Some tests or treatments are both expensive and necessary in the right situation—a balance of cost and benefit. For example, imaging and procedures may be of high value for a young patient who has lost 20 pounds unintentionally, desires a full evaluation for cancer, and is open to treatment (**Fig. 2**a). At other times, low-value care is not costly but can adversely affect quality or patient experience and even cause harm to patients. For example, a blood count laboratory test for screening in most patients is not required (**Fig. 2**b). Although the single laboratory test is not expensive by itself, the needle stick and extra time from the patient away from work at home required to collect the sample can affect patient experience. Therefore, although cost is a component of value, it does not define it.

This distinction in messaging is vital to engender engagement among patients and care teams so that they feel patients are a central priority over building revenue.[6]

IMPORTANT ROLE OF POPULATION HEALTH PROVIDERS TO CURB THE COSTS OF CARE

Since the early 2000s, traditional population health has had an emphasis in primary care to reduce variation in quality and patient experience across populations. The movement has focused on ambulatory processes and infrastructure through care delivery models such as the patient-centered medical home and the medical neighborhood. The models rely on principles of population health management (ie, access and continuity of care, comprehensiveness, plan and manage care, track and coordinate care, etc.).[7] These principles not only define major components of delivering population health but are also potential solutions to reduce expenses. The major causes of rising health care spending among populations come from hospital and physician services (**Fig. 3**).[8] For example, the average expense for

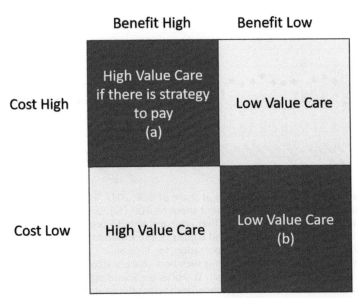

Fig. 2. Balancing costs and benefit (based on quality and patient experience). (a) If a scenario is described with high benefit and costs to pertinent stakeholders, then it would be considered a high-value service overall as long as there is a strategy to pay for the service. If a patient does not prefer to have the service, however, then it would be considered low-value care. (b) If a scenario is described with low benefit and cost to pertinent stakeholders, the service is considered low-value care.

heart failure admissions near $11,000 to 12,000 while spending on care centered out of clinic or home-based care is less expensive (near $400–500) (Medicare payment plus patient cost sharing).[9] Having a robust ambulatory infrastructure, therefore, is critical to curb expenses.

Existing models, however, have fallen short of decreasing care spending at scale thus far.[10,11] For example, the Comprehensive Primary Care initiative led by the Center for Medicare and Medicaid Innovation is one of the largest patient-centered medical home demonstrations across 7 regions. After 4 years of the program, various quality improvement outcomes improved but the program did not curb expenses over the short follow-up evaluation period. Learning from this initiative, the center has a new focus on improved efficiency within the triple aim.

Traditionally, less attention has been placed on reaching high-value care through the pathway of reducing costs and thinking about populations of patients in terms of their spending patterns. Clinicians and staff delivering population health are vital to reduce financial impacts to their health systems and patients. More affordable health care in turn may improve patient adherence, quality outcomes, and experience.

UNDERSTANDING THE COMPONENTS OF HIGH-VALUE CARE BY DIFFERENT STAKEHOLDERS
Quality Health for Populations and Patient Experience Components

Population health refers to the quality of health for patient populations that includes both health care and addresses social determinants of health. This quality is defined

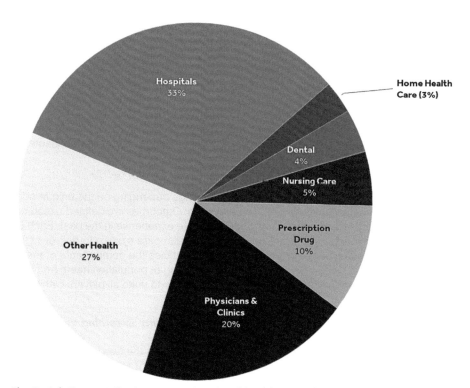

Fig. 3. Relative contributions to total national health expenditures, 2016. (*From* Kamal R, Cox C. How has U.S. spending on healthcare changed over time? Published 2017. Available at: https://www.healthsystemtracker.org/chart-collection/u-s-spending-healthcare-changed-time/#item-hospital-physician-services-represent-half-total-health-spending_2017. Accessed Nov 1, 2018.)

by the Institute of Medicine as care, to the best of current knowledge, which is safe, patient-centered, effective, efficient, timely, and equitable.[3]

In 1999, Americans learned that nearly 98,000 patients may die yearly due to preventable medical errors, which is equivalent to more than 65 titanic ships sinking.[2] The Institute of Medicine released To Err Is Human: Building a Safer Health System, an alarming report that brought public attention to the crisis of patient safety in the United States. In 2001, the Crossing the Quality Chasm: A New Health System for the 21st Century provided a more detailed examination of the enormous divide between what we know to be quality health care and the health care that people actually receive.[3] Headlines also captured the public such as when a Florida surgeon mistakenly amputated the wrong leg of a patient in 1995.

To reduce this quality chasm, medical professionals aimed to deliver evidence-based, high-quality care across patient populations. However, there are similar lost opportunities translating good practices into evidence-based medicine and ultimately into care and patient experience. In 2003, McGlynn and colleagues[12] found that only 54.9% of patients in the United States received recommended care. McGlynn's findings and newer reports from the Institute of Medicine, documenting quality and safety issues, provided focus and urgency to improve the quality of health care in the United States. There is a limitation to what evidence can truly say is of no or low value versus high value. Many things fall in the middle or vary among different patient populations. It is vital, therefore, for clinicians to know their patient population characteristics and needs. Patients and advocates also requested an improved patient experience through the health care system. As Mrs P's story describes, at the top of the article, patients' goals of care and desires could shape care planning. Chasing a diagnosis for an incidentally found nodule on imaging without eliciting Mrs P's goals can both worsen her experience and potentially create harm. Patients focus on receiving personalized care that targets what is most important to their unique situations, prior experiences, social determinants of health, and goals of care.

Understanding stakeholder perspectives

The goals of health care value have different meanings depending on the unique perspectives of members within our health care system. Outcomes are defined based on who is looking, their expectations, and what they have experience in the past. Each of these definitions provides important goals for the health care system to deliver high-value care across populations of patients. **Table 1** outlines the components of these outcomes through the lens of key stakeholders. Thinking of population heath from the patient perspective specifically, however, has the power to unite all players within the health care system.

Linkages between population health and patient experience in curbing health care costs

High-quality care is best delivered based on understanding the needs of a practice's patient population and keeping them healthy in the outpatient setting, which in return can reduce costs and improve patient experience (**Fig. 4**). Patients requiring primary preventative care such as colon cancer screening or pneumococcal vaccination have potential to reduce long-term expenses by avoiding costs related to disease. Patients with chronic conditions such as kidney disease or heart failure requiring secondary prevention have potential to avoid spending by curing or slowing down progression of disease and utilization of health care facilities and treatments. Similarly, addressing patient's social needs such as homelessness, food insecurity, or incarceration can reduce health care utilization and expenses.[13,14] Tertiary prevention or high-quality care after acute events (eg, operations, birth), anticipatory guidance, and care coordination can also reduce unnecessary facility utilization by proactively intervening on early clinical decline or patient concerns.

Financial Components

In this section the authors focus on the balance of delivering high-value care with an understanding of financial impacts of the health care system. The financial impacts can be described by total costs of care and patient affordability or out-of-pocket expenses.

In the United States, health care costs and prices are hard to predict and understand. It is, therefore, challenging to curb expenses in delivering population health without first understanding better the historical context of how the system became so complex.

The historical context of rising costs and prices

Since the turn of the twentieth century medicine looks different. Most doctors' visits previously took place in patients' homes, and charges for treatments and procedures were determined through a negotiation between the physician and patient.[14] With the widespread adoption of aseptic techniques by the 1890, people previously treated at home were now seeking treatment at hospitals.[15] In 1929, hospitals needed to recoup

Table 1
Stakeholder perspectives on pertinent outcomes and costs to achieve high-value care

Perspective	Pertinent Outcomes	Pertinent Costs
Payers/Policymakers	• High-quality, safe, equitable health care • Often focus on the aspects of population health and patient experience that is measurable through scientifically developed and rigorously standardized surveys. For example, Hospital Consumer Assessment of Healthcare Providers and Systems (HCAHPS) are often included.	• Payers focus on total costs of care across their population of beneficiaries. • Policymakers focus on the national health care GDP.
Medical center: Leadership	• High-quality, safe, equitable health care that adjusts for the complexity of the patient population.	• Total costs of care for their total patient population adjusted for the complexity of the patient population. • Defining cost-saving interventions can be challenging, because it involves balancing direct hospital costs with payment incentives and their effect on revenue and patient experience.
Medical center: Frontline clinicians and staff	• Health care that is high quality, safe, personal, equitable, and address social determinants of health. • Often emphasizes the specific measures that require reporting to payer groups.	• Total costs of care of the specific patient populations that they serve and patient's out-of-pocket expenses.
Patient/Communities	• Health care that is visibly high quality, safe, personal, equitable, and addresses social determinants of health. • Personalized care that targets what is most important to a patient's unique situation, prior experience, and goals of care. New patient-reported outcome measures (PROMs) rely on patient survey information to capture outcomes from their perspective. • Communication that is timely, convenient, and equitable with appropriate literacy levels and coordination of care from health care teams.	• Out-of-pocket expenses that can include premiums, deductibles, coinsurance, copayments, health savings and flexible health plans, and other expenses. • Currently patients face challenges in obtaining spending data at the patient level due to limitations in data transparency and with uncertainty to how to calculate accurate price estimates based on patient payment plans that can be fluid overtime.
Employers	• High-quality, safe, equitable health care that keeps employees at work and with positive experiences.	• Insurance expenses across all employee benefit plans.

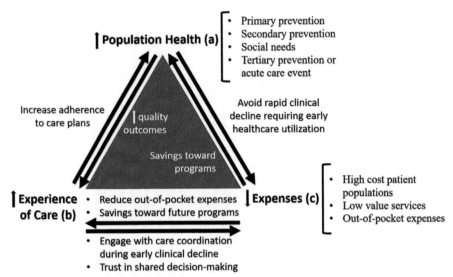

Fig. 4. Relationships between health care value components. (a) High quality of care for populations can help to reduce expenses by avoiding rapid clinical decline of patient who may benefit from preventative care or social services and improve clinical outcomes for patients. (b) Positive patient experience can also reduce expenses and improve quality of care by increasing engagement and trust in care plans aimed to reduce clinical decline. (c) Reducing health care expenses can improve patient experience by reducing out-of-pocket expenses and financial harms, and savings can be invested back into programs to improve population health and patient experience.

building and operating costs and the average annual health care charges ($67) by nearly 400% per family to $261.[16] After the world wars, medical knowledge grew, new technologies emerged, and costs increased. At this time, however, patients paid institutions directly. As the costs increased and care became more complex, price transparency disappeared.

Today, instead of having one doctor, patients can have over 20 in a short hospital stay. Medicine requires economies of scale and prices no longer rely on the patient-physician interaction. Prices are determined based on closed-door negotiations between insurance companies and provider organizations. Multiple transactions are required to deliver a single health care service, and with each exchange of dollars, there are different terms: "costs," "charges," "payments or reimbursements," and "prices." The final price, however, bears little resemblance to the original cost of production.

Defining different types of "costs" and "affordability"

"Costs" are the required expenses to provide health care services. "Charges" are the amount asked for services by health care providers. Reimbursements are the amount the payer negotiates to pay providers for rendered care (typically will be less than the charge). Prices are the amount that the patient ultimately pays for services. Patient affordability refers to the out-of-pocket expenses expected of patients. Patients frequently make purchases without knowing the prices or even fully knowing what is being sold. When the bill arrives (weeks later), as Mrs P experienced at the top of the article, it is filled with obscure information and does not reflect the original cost of creating the service (**Fig. 5**).

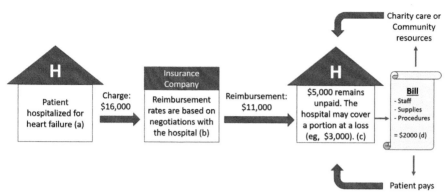

Fig. 5. Description of connection between charges, reimbursement, and prices (eg, heart failure hospitalization). (a) If a patient is hospitalized for a heart failure exacerbation, the hospital may charge the insurance company $16,000. (b) Insurance companies negotiate reimbursement rates back to the hospital; although the reimbursement amount depends on the patient's insurance plan, some will cover more or less of the expenses. (c) If the patient's insurance covers $11,000, then the remaining $5000 is billed to the patient with a portion of the price covered by the hospital as a financial loss. (d) Without insurance, however, the patient may be expected to pay a large portion of the charge themselves or apply for charity care or other community outreach to assist with their medical bills.

Understanding stakeholder perspectives

Each stakeholder in our health care system primarily views "costs" through their own lens (see **Table 1**). To health systems, relevant "costs" are the total expenses required to render services, which include variable (in the hands of clinician decision-making, eg, computed tomographic scan) and fixed costs (paid regardless of amount of care provided, eg, building lighting). Health systems also focus on charges that they request from payers to eventually compensate for the services they provided.

To payers, relevant "costs" are charges and reimbursements. Outpatient charges have been based on the number and type of visits and procedures rendered. Hospitals have charged inpatient episodes of care based on diagnosis-related condition (diagnosis-related groups) codes, which group patients with clinical problems that are expected to require similar services and resources (eg, acute on chronic systolic heart failure).[17] Medicare would reimburse hospital's standard adjusted base-payments that depend on these codes for the expenses that efficient facilities would expect.[17] For example, if Mrs Kemp (admitted for 2 days) and Mrs Jones (admitted for 10 days) received similar treatment of acute on chronic systemic heart failure, it is likely that the hospital may create savings in Mrs Kemp's case while creating a loss in Mrs Jones' case. Overtime, Medicare and other payers now emphasize accountable care payment structures that define episodes of care including both inpatient- and outpatient-based services to motivate delivering high-value, coordinated care and keeping patients well (**Fig. 6**).

To patients, relevant "costs" are prices. These expenses can include insurance premiums, deductibles, coinsurance, copayments, and health saving and flexible spending plans. Employers, similar to patients, are seeing expenses shifted to them and seek affordable health care for their institutions and employees.

Financial harms: total cost of care and patient affordability

This opaque health care system has been void of checks-and-balances for expenses that affect both our national health care system and individual patients. The United

	Fee for Service Payment	DRG Payment	Accountable Care
Reimbursement	Based on percent of gross charges, "the more we do, the more we get paid."	Based on DRG coding, does not change regardless of services performed.	Based on per member per month (PMPM) bundled payments.
In Use	Past	Present	Future
Covered Days	Some portion of days in the hospital is covered by payers.	Average reimbursement covers approximately 5 d of inpatient stay for an acute on chronic heart failure exacerbation regardless of how long the patient stays.	Not applicable- transitions to bundled payments that cover inpatient and outpatient care.
Incentive	Bill for every single supply, daily therapy consults, radiography, etc.	Accurate diagnoses and DRG coding.	Keeping people well and care coordinated to improve quality, costs, and patient experience.

Fig. 6. Difference between fee-for-service, diagnosis-related group, and accountable care payment strategies.

States leads the world in GDP health care expenditures and is projected to increase (**Fig. 7**).[18] However, with this high spending, Americans continue to perform lower in health indicators, including life expectancy, mortality and prevalence of chronic disease, and injuries.[19,20] The Institute of Medicine detailed drivers of health care waste spending and 27% ($210 billion annually) is attributed to unnecessary services. Some

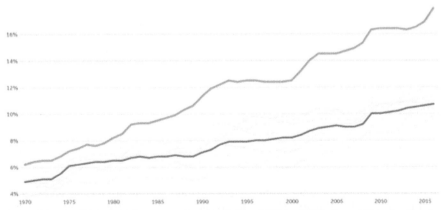

Fig. 7. Total health expenditures as percent of GDP, 1970 to 2016. Since 1980, the Gap has Widened between US Healthcare Spending and that of other countries. Green, United States; Blue, average of other OECD countries. (*From* Sawyer B, Cox C. How does health spending in the U.S. compare to other countries? Published Dec 7, 2018. Available at: https://www.healthsystemtracker.org/chart-collection/health-spending-u-s-compare-countries/#item-since-1980-gap-widened-u-s-health-spending-countries. Accessed Dec 10, 2018.)

estimates report more than 40% of services delivered to Medicare patients provide minimal clinical benefit and are thus considered low-value services.[21]

Today, everyone pays for health care with an increased shift of expenses to patient and families to pick up the burden of costs. The percent of adults on high-deductible plans has increased from 26.3% in 2011 to 39.3% in 2016, and the average plan deductible exceeds a typical family's available savings.[22] The Kaiser Family Foundation reports that patient annual contributions for insurance premiums has increased by nearly 30% from both employers and patients and projected annual family health care expenses (premium plus out-of-pocket expenses) are increasing exponentially.[23]

Medical bills are the leading cause of all financial harms to patients by placing a burden on their disposable incomes and can potentially lead to bankruptcy.[24] For services that are not covered under an insurance policy, patients are left paying inflated prices. A pivotal manuscript, Do No (Financial) Harm, shared that a single health care decision will create a ripple effect of expenses including further workup and opportunity costs such as foregone wages causing thousands of dollars of out-of-pocket expenses as experienced by Mrs P at the top of the article.[25] A Kaiser Family Foundation survey highlighted how these impacts on out-of-pocket expenses may affect the quality and experience of health care that patients receive. Over 50% of patients surveyed reported doing at least one of the activities described in **Fig. 8**, including skipping recommended tests or treatments, over the last 12 months due to healthcare costs.[25]

Not surprisingly, patient would like to openly discuss the prices of their health care with their clinicians (two-thirds of patients in multisite study surveyed).[26] When conversations do occur, patient report better experience even if they do not receive initially requested tests or treatments and conversations often change management plans.[27] These conversations, however, are occurring less than 15% to 20% of the time.[26]

Linkages between reducing costs of health care with population health and patient experience

Having parallel efforts to both reduce total costs of care and improve patient affordability can help improve population health and patient experience goals. Savings from reducing total costs of care can create revenue to redirect toward population health programs. Similarly, avoiding financial harms to patient can improve patient experience. It can also lead to improved adherence to outpatient appointments and medications that maintain high-quality care out of the hospital with 13% of

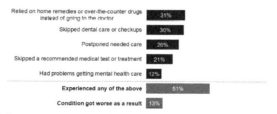

Fig. 8. Half of adults report putting off care due to costs; some say their conditions got worse as a result of skipping care. Prompt: Percent who say they or someone else in their household did each of the following in the past 12 months because of the cost. (*From* From Kirzinger A, Muñana C, Wu B, et al. Data note: Americans' challenges with health care costs. Available at: https://www.kff.org/health-costs/issue-brief/data-note-americans-challenges-health-care-costs/. Published Jun 11, 2019; with permission.)

American adults reporting that their condition worsened as a result of healthcare costs.[23,25]

OPPORTUNITIES TO IMPROVE HIGH-VALUE CARE THROUGH POPULATION HEALTH AND REDUCING THE COSTS OF CARE
For Policy Makers and Payers

Initial motivations for change led to new policies with performance incentives to guide health systems to reach the triple aim. Government policy promoted high-value care by mandating data collection using scientifically developed and standardized surveys, linking payment incentives to these new metrics, and publicly reporting provider performance (**Table 2** for detailed examples).

Financial incentives

For decades health systems have been paid through a fee-for-service billing model, which reimburses and incentivizes providers to test, treat, visit, code, and bill for more.[28] The fee-for-service model, unfortunately, has been associated with poor quality care, including delayed diagnoses, complications, readmissions, increased length of stay, and high costs of care.[28]

With trying to pack more into a day, primary care has seen high volumes of short clinic visits and increasing workforce burnout. With these concerns, the United States is projected to face a shortage of between 40,800 and 104,900 physicians by 2030.[29] Deemphasizing ambulatory care can limit solutions to produce high-value care such as outpatient care coordination, less expensive ambulatory sites of care, and development of care pathways. For example, traditionally primary care duties that could prevent more expensive facility utilization such as out-of-clinic visit calls, emails, prescription refills, and reviewing laboratories and imaging have not been reimbursed.[30]

As a result, the Centers of Medicare and Medicaid Services has introduced new payment models that tie quality and value incentives to 90% of fee-for-service payments and provide 50% of Medicare payments through alternative payment models.[31] Medicaid and other commercial payers followed suit. These models, instead, hold health systems accountable through risk-based financial contracts that could potentially lead to financial losses if they do not reach performance outcomes among the patient population they serve. The models increase freedom to creatively and efficiently redesign care delivery and emphasize improving ambulatory care systems.

Providing performance transparency to the public

In the early 2000s, there was significant variability in health system quality and increasing charges to payers compared with the costs for rendered care, thus inflating prices.[32] However, new user-friendly, online tools and policies have promoted putting performance information and prices into the hands of the public. Athough these tools are not perfect and continue to be improved, the information can help consumers make informed decisions about where to go for high-quality, less costly health care and help curb variation in quality and some costs.

For Health Systems, Practitioners, and Staff

Health systems have an overwhelming responsibility to translate new policies into interventions that improve the triple aim among their patient populations. Redesigning care to meet these goals will require strategies codeveloped with care teams, patients, and visible leaders to identify areas of opportunity and build a pipeline of trained clinicians and staff and infrastructure to delivery high-value care. Reducing expenses can

Table 2
Opportunities to improve high-value care

Stakeholder	Opportunities	Sub-opportunities	Examples
Payers	Using financial incentives	Models to promote robust ambulatory infrastructure to keep patients healthy and out of the hospital.	Models include the Pioneer Accountable Care Organizations (ACOs), Next Generation ACOs, Comprehensive Primary Care initiatives, End Stage Renal Disease, and others. (https://innovation.cms.gov/initiatives/index.html#views=models)
		Models encouraging investing savings back into patient or community programs.	Accountable Health Communities (https://innovation.cms.gov/initiatives/ahcm/)
		Models of insurance design to incentive patients directly by reducing out-of-pocket expenses for high-value care.	Adherence to chronic diabetes medications increased by 7%–14% when patient copays were reduced compared to control groups.[38]
	Increasing pubic transparency	Developing consumer-oriented website that provides information on how hospitals provide recommended care to patients.	Hospital Compare was developed by Medicare and Hospital Quality Alliance.[39]
			For a common heart failure admission in 2012, Seattle healthcare centers submitted charges ranging between $8900 and $21,000. While some medical centers received different reimbursement for these cases based on their negotiated contracts, this disparity closed over time with continued public transparency.[39]
		Expanding payer-provider partnerships to better inform patients about expenses at the point-of-care.	When customers with Blue Cross North Carolina select high-value services such as a lower-cost care site to obtain a $1000 MRI, they are mailed $200. (Conversation with Patrick H. Conway, President and CEO of Blue Cross Blue Shield of North Carolina, September 13, 2018.)
			Medicare is similarly promoting price transparency and patient counseling about billing.[40]

(continued on next page)

Table 2
(continued)

Stakeholder	Opportunities	Sub-opportunities	Examples
Medical centers and practices	Reducing population-based expenses	Identifying patients with chronic conditions and acute care episodes of care driving expenses locally.	The University of California Los Angeles (UCLA) Health, implemented a system-wide approach to identify patient populations with high expenses including:
			for example, chronic conditions: cancer, chronic kidney disease, and dementia, mental health
			for example, acute care episodes of care: knee and hip surgeries
		Developing care pathways for each risk tier.	The top 1% of patients (22% expenditures) received intensive multi-specialty, multi-interdisciplinary care coordination and palliative care. UCLA believed addressing only the most expensive 1% of patients alone may not reduce spending since patients with complex medical and social needs require significant resources and this strategy would focus on individual patients rather than populations.[35]
			The middle 19% of patients (58% expenditures) received increasing levels of care coordination, community resources, and advanced care planning.[41]
			The bottom 80% of patients (20% expenditures) require healthcare screening, condition-specific prevention, and reduction of unnecessary care to reduce long-term costs.[40]
	Reducing low value care	Reducing high-cost low-volume services	Knee arthroscopy
		Reducing high-volume low unit cost services	Complete blood count laboratory test
		Addressing cultural barriers to de-implementation	The High Value Care Culture Survey (HVCCS™) measures culture to addressing these barriers in designing local interventions. (http://www.highvaluecarecultures urvey.com/)
	Reducing out-of-pocket expenses	Improving price transparency to patients	University of Utah created the Pricing Transparency tool that, with patient inputs about their health plan deductible or co-payments, provides estimates of out-of-pocket expenses for common procedures. (https://healthcare.utah.edu/pricing/)

Engaging, training, and developing networks of clinicians and staff who discuss costs

Access data at the point-of-care and incorporate it into care plans
- Screening patients
- Connect patients with financial counselors or community resources addressing social needs
- Patient billing improvement

Costs of Care Inc., a global NGO that develops and disseminates innovations in high-value care, has developed initial guides, educational modules, and provider training focused on cost conversations and affordability. (https://costsofcare.org/)

Care team can elicit the needs of their patient population and identify which subpopulations are at greater risk of financial harms.

Groups such as Health Leads link patients to essential resources like food, housing and transportation alongside medical care within communities. (https://healthleadsusa.org/)

CareMore addresses patient transportation barriers by contracting with on-demand transportation companies. (https://www.caremore.com/Home/About/News/2018/20180913-Health-Affairs.aspx)

UCLA's billing office have focused on improving patient experience by reducing call wait times to reach a live person who can provide situation-specific information. (Conversation with Anton Loman, Director, UCLA Patient Billing Office, December 4, 2018.)

(continued on next page)

Table 2
(continued)

Stakeholder	Opportunities	Sub-opportunities	Examples
Patients	Co-develop programs	Consumer-directed policies, insurance design, and local improvement efforts	University of Utah determined some of their system-wide value-improvement initiatives based on patient input such as reducing clinic wait times through a design studio model. (https://uofuhealth.utah.edu/accelerate/blog/2018/08/marcie-hopkins-university-of-utah-health-patient-design-studio-what-do-patients-want-ask-them.php)
	Co-develop patient-facing tools	Shared decision-making tools	Mayo Clinic and Kaiser Permanente have created a national shared-decision making resource centers. (https://shareddecisions.mayoclinic.org/)
	Sharing experiences	–	Costs of Care Inc. has curated over 500 patient stories outlining the financial impact to patients from care decisions and has extracted and collated key areas of improvement opportunity. (https://costsofcare.org/annual-story-contest/)
	Developing networks	–	Cancer Care, which focuses on patients with cancer, has developed website networks where patients and families can ask questions and gain time care, education, and financial assistance. (https://www.cancercare.org/)
Employers	Internal hiring	–	Apple and Amazon hired their own clinicians and use technology to deliver more efficient care. (https://www.forbes.com/sites/brucejapsen/2018/08/17/amazons-clinics-join-employer-push-into-worksite-healthcare/#500afafa3ace)
	Contracting	–	Boeing aligned with Mayo Clinic rather than local medical center to offer certain orthopeadic surgeries in order to provide more affordable, high quality care to their employees. (https://www.mayoclinic.org/centers-of-excellence/boeing)
	Using efficient tools and technology	–	RowdMap's Risk-Readiness Benchmarks can help identify, quantify, and reduce low-value care that clinicians deliver and where their patients could receive higher value healthcare. (https://rowdmap.com/)

be organized into 3 major areas: reducing population-based spending, low-value care, and patient out-of-pocket expenses (see **Table 2**).

Reducing population-based spending

Current care fragmentation and operational inefficiencies are associated with poorly co-ordinated, duplicated, and varied care.[8,33] For example, Yarnall and colleagues found that it would take primary care providers 21 hours a day to delivery chronic, acute, and preventative care to their patients on any given day. In reality, however, they only have 1.3 hours a day to focus on preventative care.[34] Without time allocation toward these efforts and infrastructure to coordinate management between primary, specialty, and inpatient care, disease progression and potential health care utilization can ensue. Therefore, health systems can aim to identify patient subpopulations with high expenses, organize them into risk tiers incorporating expenses and utilization, and promote proactive value-based care. They can develop interventions and care pathways that address patients' needs at each risk tier to achieve short- and long-term savings.[35]

Reducing low-value care

Low- or no-value services are those that provide no net health benefit in specific clinical scenarios. These services include those that are high cost (eg, knee arthroscopy) and high volume with low unit costs (eg, laboratory tests) with the latter driving more unnecessary spending.[36] Success of efforts to reduce these low-value services will depend on tactics to deimplement, or unlearn, practice tradition and create a high-value care culture.

Reducing patient out-of-pocket expenses

Although reducing unnecessary care is required to curb expenses, there are situations when care is both necessary and expensive. Developing systems to support these scenarios can also improve patient out-of-pocket expenses and experiences. Health systems can focus on providing actionable price transparency to patients, train and shift care to care teams that can deliver affordable care, and develop care pathways to support patients vulnerable to financial risks. Additionally, different sources of low value health care costs account for higher out-of-pocket costs (e.g. durable medical equipment) compared to health system costs (e.g. hospital care).[37]

For Patients

Patients have advocated for increased affordable health care through codeveloping programs and patient-facing tools with health systems, payers, and policymakers. Patients have organized to share their experiences and create networks to support each other through expensive care episodes (see **Table 2**).

For Employers

Employers who often fund the bill for their employees' health care have also focused on purchasing higher-value health care. They are hiring internal clinicians, contracting with high-value providers, and using more patient-friendly tools to coordinate care (see **Table 2**).

SUMMARY

The US health care system is complex with inefficiencies, and the public has asked for increased health care quality and experience with reduced expenses. With many stakeholders involved in improving health care value for populations, it will be important to understand how health care value is defined and appropriately messaged to improve outcomes for each group. Providers of population health have a vital role to achieve these goals. By delivering coordinated, evidence-based primary, secondary, tertiary prevention and addressing social needs, providers can help patients stay healthy longer and out of the hospital. In-return, improving the affordability of health care for patients is associated with improved adherence to care, maintenance of high-quality care out of the hospital, and patient experience. Similarly, savings from these efforts can continue to fund future improvement interventions.

Understanding these relationships can identify improvement opportunities for policy makers, health systems, patients, and employers. Improvement will, however, require thinking beyond metrics and payer-based programs alone and moving toward broader programs that will create health for patient populations across our health care systems.

REFERENCES

1. The Institute for Healthcare Improvement (IHI). Available at: http://www.ihi.org/Topics/TripleAim/Pages/default.aspx. Accessed November 25, 2018.
2. Kohn LT, Corrigan JM, Donaldson MS. To err is human: building a safer health system. Washington, DC: Institute of Medicine; National Academy Press; 2000.
3. Institute of Medicine. Crossing the quality chasm: a new health system for the 21st century. Washington, DC: National Academy Press; 2001.
4. Mueller M, Morgan D. OECD health statistics. In: Spending on health latest trends. 2018. Available at: http://www.oecd.org/health/health-systems/Health-Spending-Latest-Trends-Brief.pdf. Accessed November 1, 2018.
5. Porter ME. What is value in health care? N Engl J Med 2010;363:2477–81.
6. Liao JM, Schapira MS, Navathe AS, et al. The effect of emphasizing patient, societal, and institutional harms of inappropriate antibiotic prescribing on physician support of financial penalties: a randomized trial. Ann Intern Med 2017;167:215–6.
7. Huang X, Rosenthal MB. Transforming specialty practice- the patient-centered medical neighborhood. N Engl J Med 2014;370(75):1376–9.
8. The Henry J. Kaiser Family Foundation analysis of National Health Expenditure (NHE) data from Centers for Medicare and Medicaid Services, Office of the Actuary, National Health Statistics Group (2017). 2017. Available at: https://www.healthsystemtracker.org/chart-collection/u-s-spending-healthcare-changed-time/#item-hospital-physician-services-represent-half-total-health-spending_2017. Accessed November 1, 2018.
9. Fitch K, Engel T, Lau J. The cost burden of worsening heart failure in the medicare fee for service population: an actuarial analysis. Milliman report. 2017. Available at: http://us.milliman.com/uploadedFiles/insight/2017/cost-bruden-worsening-heart-failure.pdf. Accessed November 1, 2018.
10. Congressional Budget Office. Lessons from Medicare's demonstration projects on disease management, care coordination, and value-based payment. Washington, DC: CBO; 2012. Available at: http://www.cbo.gov/sites/default/files/cbofiles/attachments/01-18-12-MedicareDemoBrief.pdf.
11. Peikes D, Dale S, Ghosh A, et al. The comprehensive primary care initiative: effects on spending, quality, patients, and physicians. Health Aff (Millwood) 2018;37(6):890–9.
12. McGlynn EA, Asch SM, Adams J, et al. The quality of health care delivered to adults in the United States. N Engl J Med 2003;348:2635–45.

13. Kushel MB, Gupta R, Gee L, et al. Housing instability and food insecurity as barriers to health care among low-income Americans. J Gen Intern Med 2006; 21(1):71–7.

14. Wang EA, Wang Y, Krumholz HM. A high risk of hospitalization following release from correctional facilities in medicare beneficiaries: a retrospective matched cohort study, 2002-2010. JAMA Intern Med 2013;173(17):1621–8.

15. Rosenberg CE. The care of strangers: the rise of America's hospital system. Baltimore (MD): Johns Hopkins University Press; 1987.

16. Gorman L. The history of health care costs and health insurance. Wisconsin Policy Research Institute Report, vol. 19, 2006 (10):1–31. Available at: http://www.wpri.org/WPRI-Files/Special-Reports/Reports-Documents/Vol19no10.pdf. Accessed September 10, 2015.

17. MedPAC. Hospital acute inpatient services payment system. 2015. Available at: http://www.medpac.gov/docs/default-source/payment-basics/hospital-acute-inpatient-services-payment-system-15.pdf?sfvrsn=0. Accessed November 1, 2018.

18. Sawyer B, Cox C. The Henry J. Kaiser Family Foundation analysis of National Health Expenditure (NHE) data from Centers for Medicare and Medicaid Services, Office of the Actuary, National Health Statistics Group. (2017), "How does health spending in the U.S. compare to other countries?". 2018. Available at: https://www.healthsystemtracker.org/chart-collection/health-spending-u-s-compare-countries/#item-since-1980-gap-widened-u-s-health-spending-countries. Accessed December 10, 2018.

19. OECD Health Statistics 2017. Life expectancy at birth and health spending per capita, 2015. 2017. Available at: https://www.oecd-ilibrary.org/docserver/health_glance-2017-6-en.pdf?expires=1543783820&id=id&accname=guest&checksum=8FB8EF9EC254A57B267E565ABE3F1BA5. Accessed November 1, 2018.

20. Squires D, Anderson C. U.S. Health Care from a Global Perspective: Spending, Use of Services, Prices, and Health in 13 Countries. The Commonwealth Fund: Issues in International Health Policy. 2015. Available at: http://www.commonwealthfund.org/publications/issue-briefs/2015/oct/us-health-care-from-a-global-perspective. Accessed November 1, 2018.

21. Schwartz AL, Landon BE, Elshaug AG, et al. Measuring low-value care in medicare. JAMA Intern Med 2014;174(7):1067–76.

22. Cohen RA, Zammiti EP. High-deductible health plans and financial Barriers to medical care: early Release of estimates from the national health Interview survey, 2016. Centers of Disease Control: National Center for Health Statistics. 2017. Available at: https://www.cdc.gov/nchs/data/nhis/earlyrelease/ERHDHP_Access_0617.pdf. Accessed November 1, 2018.

23. Kaiser Family Foundation. 2016 Employer health benefits survey. 2016. Available at: https://www.kff.org/report-section/ehbs-2016-summary-of-findings/. Accessed November 1, 2018.

24. Moriates C, Shah NT, Arora VM. First, do no (financial) harm. JAMA 2013;310(6): 577–8.

25. Kirzinger A, Muñana C, Wu B, et al. Data note: Americans' challenges with health care costs. The Henry J. Kaiser Family Foundation; 2019. KFF Health Tracking Poll (conducted March 13-18, 2019). Available at: https://www.kff.org/health-costs/issue-brief/data-note-americans-challenges-health-care-costs/. Accessed July 1, 2019.

26. Alexander CG, Casalino LP, Tseng CW, et al. Barriers to patient-physician communication about out-of-pocket costs. J Gen Intern Med 2014;19(8):856–60.
27. Tipirneni R, Patel MR, Kirch MA, et al. Cost conversations between primary care providers and patients with expanded medicaid coverage. J Gen Intern Med 2018;33(11):1845–7.
28. Miller HD. From volume to value: better way to pay for health care. Health Aff 2009;28(5):1418–28.
29. Mann S. Research Shows shortage of more than 100,000 doctors by 2030. AAMC news 2017. Available at: https://news.aamc.org/medical-education/article/new-aamc-research-reaffirms-looming-physician-shor/. Accessed November 1, 2018.
30. Baron RJ. What's keeping us so busy in primary care? A snapshot from one practice. N Engl J Med 2010;362(17):1632–6.
31. Burwell SM. Setting value-based payment goals-HHS efforts to improve U.S. Health care. N Engl J Med 2015;372(10):897–9.
32. National Nurses United. New Data - Some Hospitals Set Charges at 10 Times their Costs. 2014. Available at: https://www.nationalnursesunited.org/press/new-data-some-hospitals-set-charges-10-times-their-costs. Accessed November 1, 2018.
33. Kern LM, Seirup JK, Rajan M, et al. Fragmented ambulatory care and subsequent healthcare utilization among medicare beneficiaries. Am J Manag Care 2018; 24(9):294–300.
34. Yarnell KSH, Ostbye T, Krause KM, et al. Family physicians as team leaders: "time" to share the care. Prev Chronic Dis 2009;6(2):A59.
35. McWilliams JM, Schwartz AL. Focusing on high-cost patients—the key to addressing high costs? N Engl J Med 2018;376(9):807–9.
36. Mafi JM, RussellK, Bortz BA, et al. Low-cost, high-volume health services contribute the most to unnecessary health spending. Health Aff 2017;36(10): 1701–4.
37. Personal Health Expenditures by Expenditure Type and Source of Funds in 2017. Centers for Medicare and Medicaid Services. Office of the Actuary, National Health Statistics Group. National Health Expenditure Accounts (NHEA). NHE tables ZIP file: Table 4 year 2017. Available at: https://www.cms.gov/research-statistics-data-and-systems/statistics-trends-and-reports/nationalhealthexpenddata/natio nalhealthaccountshistorical.html. Accessed August 1, 2019.
38. Chernew ME, Shah M, Wegh A, et al. Impact of decreasing copayments on medication adherence within a disease management environment. Health Aff 2006; 27(1):103–12.
39. Centers for Medicare and Medicaid Services. Hospital Compare. 2016. Available at: https://www.cms.gov/medicare/quality-initiatives-patient-assessment-instrum ents/hospitalqualityinits/hospitalcompare.html. Accessed November 1, 2018.
40. Federal Register Proposed Rule Doc. 2018-08705. Medicare Programs: Hospital Inpatient Prospective Payment Systems for Acute Care Hospitals and Long Term Care Hospital Prospective Payment System and Proposed Policy Changes and Fiscal Year 2019 Rates; etc. Centers for Medicare and Medicaid Services. 2018. Available at: https://www.federalregister.gov/documents/2018/05/07/2018-08705/medicare-programs-hospital-inpatient-prospective-payment-systems-for-acute-care-hospitals-and-long. Accessed November 1, 2018.
41. Gupta R, Roh L, Lee C, et al. The Population Health Value Framework. Creating Value by Reducing Costs of Care for Patient Subpopulations With Chronic Conditions. Acad Med 2019;94(9):1337–42.

The Business Case for Population Health Management

Jason H. Wasfy, MD, MPhil[a,b,*], Timothy G. Ferris, MD, MPH[b,c]

KEYWORDS

• Health policy • Accountable care organizations • Population health management

KEY POINTS

• As payments for health care transition from fee-for-service to value-based, health care providers have been described as operating "in two canoes." In the fee-for-service canoe, providers have incentives to provide more frequent and more expensive services. At the same time, in the value-based payment canoe, providers have incentives to reduce inappropriate and unhelpful utilization of health care.

• We believe that the business case to develop culture, business practice, and infrastructure for value-based care is strong for several reasons.

• These clinical examples represent straightforward ways to succeed in a "mixed-payer" environment, where population health programs coexist with programs meant to generate external referrals.

INTRODUCTION

As payments for health care transition from fee-for-service to value-based payments, health care providers have been described as operating "in two canoes." In the fee-for-service canoe, providers have incentives to provide more frequent and more expensive services. At the same time, in the value-based payment canoe, providers have incentives to reduce inappropriate and unhelpful utilization of health care.[1] At first glance, traveling in these two canoes at the same time may seem perilous. Both the

Disclosures: Dr J.H. Wasfy reports serving on the Learning and Action Network Committee on Episode-Based Payment for Cardiac Conditions (unpaid) and as vice-chair of the New England Comparative Effectiveness Public Advisory Council. He also reports grant support from the National Institutes of Health through Harvard Catalyst (KL2 TR001100) and from the American Heart Association (18CDA34110215).

a Cardiology Division, Department of Medicine, Massachusetts General Hospital, Harvard Medical School, Boston, MA, USA; b Massachusetts General Physicians Organization, Harvard Medical School, Boston, MA, USA; c Department of Medicine, Massachusetts General Hospital, Harvard Medical School, Boston, MA, USA
* Corresponding author. Massachusetts General Physicians Organization, 55 Fruit Street, Boston, MA 02114.
E-mail address: jwasfy@mgh.harvard.edu

Prim Care Clin Office Pract 46 (2019) 623–629
https://doi.org/10.1016/j.pop.2019.07.003
primarycare.theclinics.com

clinical infrastructure and the clinical culture required for success at these different goals are likely to be different.

This "two canoes" mixed-payment system also carries important implications for health care providers and the health care system nationally. First, risk contracts force providers to actively weigh volume and income aspirations with broader societal benefits and the need to achieve a sustainable cost growth rate nationally. Second, these contracts attempt to transfer the pursuit of important societal goals to health care provider organizations. Unfortunately, there is no payment system that can perfectly align what patients need with what contracts reimburse.

We believe that the business case to develop culture, business practice, and infrastructure for value-based care is strong for several reasons. First, in some ways, value-based care can improve margins in fee-for-service contracts even while it also reduces costs for local populations. For example, encouraging shared-decision making with patients about joint arthroplasty could reduce unwarranted expenditures in a local population while also creating more operating room capacity for external referrals. This type of shift would improve a hospital's performance in contracts that involve shared financial risk but also potentially improve hospital margin in fee-for-service business. Importantly, it could improve the quality of care for both populations, particularly if hospital capacity is already constrained.

Similarly, improving care coordination and transitions to outpatient care for patients with percutaneous coronary intervention[2] can reduce the cost of care for patients receiving routine percutaneous coronary intervention by reducing hospital readmissions. At the same time, these avoided readmissions can lead to more inpatient bed availability to allow the development of advanced techniques, such as transcatheter valve replacement, that attract patients from outside the local region.

These clinical examples represent straightforward ways to succeed in a mixed-payer environment, where population health programs coexist with programs meant to generate external referrals. In principle, decisions could be more difficult when these tradeoffs are more stark (eg, in program development). Complex care management programs[3] are unlikely to improve margin in fee-for-service. Furthermore, changes in public policy may cause uncertainty about the pace and form of transitions in payment policy.[4]

With these more difficult decisions about organizational priorities, however, we believe that although the pace and form of a transition to value-based payment are uncertain, the end result is much clearer. Simply put, the persistent rise in the cost of health care in America is unsustainable. Furthermore, public pressure is likely to demand a health care system that produces better clinical outcomes.

HEALTH CARE COSTS AND THE US ECONOMY: IMPLICATIONS FOR LONG-TERM PROVIDER STRATEGY

In 2016, health care accounted for 17.9% of the total gross domestic product (GDP) of the United States, an amount equivalent to $10,348 per person.[5] In 1960, health care accounted for only 5.0% of GDP.[6] Over that time period, therefore, the proportion of health care costs within the overall economy has more than tripled. This proportion differs markedly from the proportion in other countries. For example, health care accounts for 9.6% of the GDP in Australia, 10.3% in Canada, and 11.9% in Sweden.[7]

Although the outlier status of the United States is clear in terms of proportion of the overall economy spent on health care, the contributing factors to that outlier status on other aspects of the economy is less clear. Conceptually, high health care costs could decrease the profitability of businesses that pay for employees' insurance and even encourage them to employ fewer people, raising unemployment, or decrease wages. Another concern is that increased costs borne by states could cause direct reductions in spending on other public priorities, such as education, housing, or public security. Although these concerns are conceptually valid, little rigorous evidence exists to demonstrate that higher health care costs have a deleterious effect on other aspects of the economy.[8]

Despite the lack of rigorous evidence, anecdotal evidence cited in the popular media commonly attribute economic problems to health care costs.[8] Furthermore, to the extent that individual patients bear the direct burden of health care costs, there is an association between substantial household financial burden and illness. For example, one in four low-income families in which one member has atherosclerotic cardiovascular disease experiences out of pocket medical expenses that exceed 20% of the household budget.[9] For these reasons, public pressure for providers to reduce the cost of care seems likely to persist.

Generally, the high aggregate spending on health care is related to higher costs and higher utilization of health care, in addition to population growth and aging.[10] In addition, changes in disease prevalence and incidence seem to be reducing the overall cost of care.[10] Some excess costs seem to be related to a greater intensity of delivery of services. For example, among the Organization for Economic Co-operation and Development (OECD) countries, the United States ranks 6 out of 11 in the incidence of myocardial infarction (192 per 100,000 population per year).[7] However, the highest number of coronary artery bypass surgeries are performed (79 per 100,000 population per year) and the second-highest number of percutaneous coronary intervention are performed (248 per 100,000 population per year) in the United States.[7] For coronary disease in the United States, the intensity of procedures and surgery exceed the population-adjusted incidence of disease.

The greater contributor to excess spending, however, seems to be high wages and prices among doctors, nurses, and other health care professionals rather than high intensity of services. For example, specialist physicians make 5.3 times the average wage and generalist physicians make 3.6 times the average wage in the United States, ratios higher than any other OECD country.[7] Pharmaceutical spending is about double the average in these other countries.[7] Provider organization administrative costs are also much higher in the United States than other comparable countries.[7]

Establishing a coherent provider organizational strategy in the setting of changing policy priorities may seem difficult. Different public priorities and approaches may shift incentives in the short and even medium term. However, in the broad setting of American health economics and policy, any long-term organizational strategy seems much clearer. Given the high costs and mediocre outcomes of health care, long-term pressure and incentives to reduce costs are likely to persist and even accelerate.

In principle, American health care costs could be brought closer to the costs of other countries with either reduction in prices or reduction in utilization. Reduction in prices has conceptual problems, including reduction in the incentives to invest in research and development (pharmaceutical) and reduction in the incentives for talented individuals to pursue careers in health care (wages). Given the volatility of margins of health care provider organizations, reductions in prices could produce disruptive immediate effects in health care delivery and access.

In the setting of these drawbacks of reducing prices, provider organizations choosing to respond to the long-term rise in health care costs could shift infrastructure and patterns of care to engage in reductions in utilization through population health management. Reduction in utilization of effective services could reduce costs, but would violate the basic mission of health care providers and provider organizations to improve health. A long-term shift to population health management is the clearest and surest business response to these long-term structural challenges in American medicine. Although the short-term policies may shift, the long-term structural incentives to provide high-value health care will not.

EXISTING BUSINESS PRESSURES ON HEALTH CARE PROVIDERS

Responding to these long-term incentives to shift toward value-oriented care is difficult, because of the existing financial pressures on provider organizations. We believe that decreased financial pressure on hospitals and doctors related to expansion of insurance during implementation of the Affordable Care Act may allow more flexibility to invest in value-oriented infrastructure and programs. Furthermore, the introduction of new programs and contracts, including accountable care organizations (ACOs), offer the opportunity for funds that could support infrastructure and programs that could improve value over time.

In states that expanded Medicaid programs under the Affordable Care Act, hospitals have experienced increased Medicaid revenue, decreased uncompensated care costs, and improvement in profit margins.[11] Furthermore, the proportion of US hospitals with negative operating and total margins has been steadily decreasing since 2000.[12] In 2016, the aggregate total hospital margin for community hospitals was 7.8%, higher than 4.2% in 2001.[12] Although hospital margins vary based on type of hospital and region,[13] these results suggest that hospitals may have more financial bandwidth currently than in the past to invest in expensive infrastructure and programs than they did in previous years. In addition, features of evolving payment models, including shared savings in ACOs, may provide additional revenue to support this type of work. We believe that upfront availability of funds is critical for a transition to value-based care, because clinical culture and infrastructure will likely take many years to develop before improvements in quality and coordination cause reductions in the growth of cost of care.

REPUTATIONAL AND MISSION-DRIVEN ADVANTAGES TO PROVIDERS OF VALUE-ORIENTED CARE

Public attention is focused on the high costs and variable quality of care currently delivered. As such, even without full risk incentives for all patients, programs that improve value may improve the public perception of providers and health systems. In fact, leaders of health plans and health systems cite the value of the care delivered by or coordinated by their organizations.[14,15] These type of public statements underscore the degree to which values has become part of provider reputation, even before any transition to full risk-oriented contracting. "Persisting with an outdated model ultimately may lead to unacceptably high financial and public-relations costs, as payers shift their business to higher-value competitors whose approaches to care are perceived as more responsible and sustainable."[16]

Furthermore, as mission-driven organizations, hospitals, physician groups, and other providers may find that addressing the unsustainable rises in the cost of care are part of their mission to serve local communities. Health care provider organizations can function as a public trust, with community service as core elements of their missions. At the Massachusetts General Hospital, improving "the health and well-being of the diverse communities we serve" is part of the mission statement.[17] At UCLA Health System, community engagement is a core part of the institutional mission.[18] Many health care providers and other employees of provider organizations have chosen careers in health care because of an interest in serving communities. Inefficient and ineffective health care delivery affect not only the health of communities but also the financial welfare of communities, through costs imposed on local governments, businesses, and directly to patients. In that context, even before stronger financial incentives emerge, population health management may serve the community service mission of provider organizations.

FINANCIAL ADVANTAGES TO PROVIDERS OF VALUE-ORIENTED CARE

In addition to preparing for more financial risk, substantial financial advantages already exist for providers to pursue value in care delivery. In 2005, Centers for Medicare & Medicaid Services selected six organizations for a 3-year demonstration project intended to incentivize better coordination of care.[19] This Care Management for High Cost Beneficiaries demonstration tested the hypothesis that better coordination of care could improve health outcomes and reduce costs for Medicare patients with complex medical needs.[19] From this early experience, larger programs have emerged within Medicare. In particular, the Affordable Care Act of 2010 introduced Medicare ACOs, and 32 providers were selected as the original Pioneer ACOs in 2011.[20] Assessment on financial performance began on January 1, 2012, and the program was concluded at the end of 2016, with nine ACOs still participating.[20]

ACOs have become more numerous and covered more patients over time. In 2018, more than 1000 ACOs representing nearly 1500 ACO contracts exist throughout the United States.[21] They include private insurance companies and Medicare and Medicaid. In this context, now about 40 million Americans are covered by an insurance plan attributable to an ACO.[21]

In addition, other changes in payment policy continue to shift business incentives for provider organizations. Previously, the Balanced Budget Act of 1997 established the sustainable growth rate (SGR). The SGR was a method that would restrict the total growth in the cost of health care for Medicare beneficiaries to total growth in the overall US economy, and other factors including the number of fee-for-service Medicare beneficiaries, and changes in expenditures because of changes in laws and regulations. Health care inflation rising faster than overall inflation had the effect of repeated recommendations of cuts in physicians' fees. Only once, however, did those actual recommendations result in a cut, in 2002.[22] Instead, repeated threats of cuts caused planning difficulties among individual doctors and provider organizations. The SGR effectively preserved a fee-for-service backbone to Medicare payment policy, while costs continued to rise and long-term accounting for Medicare did not reflect the "doc fixes" that Congress would commonly pass to avoid SGR recommendations from coming into effect.

The SGR was repealed by the 2015 Medicare Access and CHIP Reauthorization Act (MACRA). In addition to repealing the SGR, MACRA shifted this backbone of Medicare payment to a value-oriented system. In effect, MACRA replaced a method that called for repeated cuts in physicians' fees but retained the underlying fee-for-service system with a value-based system. In that sense, the replacement of SGR with MACRA conceptually demonstrates the business incentives for providers. Given the long-term structural issues with health care costs and the American economy, there is an inevitable tradeoff: rate reductions or a shift to value-oriented payment.

In addition to crystalizing that conceptual tradeoff, MACRA also brought to health care providers more incentives to invest in value-oriented care. Consistent with the modest early success of ACOs is the concept that infrastructure investments and clinical culture will take years to effectively transform. As such, the long-term prospect of increasing value-based contractual arrangements and providers holding more risk should motivate value-based case. But ACOs have already grown nationally, covering nearly 40 million patients. Furthermore, with the implementation of MACRA, the underlying structure of Medicare payment already incentivizes value-oriented care. Since there are really only two options for creating sustainable costs in healthcare, price cuts or managing services, and ACO experience to date suggests that ACOs can successfully slow the rate of cost growth, then we should use this evidence to double down on ACO/population health approach using cost growth targets and modest downside incentives. In the short term, decreasing the high US administrative costs would provide significant headroom to pay for the necessary infrastructure investments without increasing overall costs. In short, providing ineffective or inappropriate care is not sound long-term business strategy, and modest value based payment incentives create a business case to manage these excesses when and where they occur.

SUMMARY

At first glance, business incentives for health care organizations seem complex as payment systems transition from fee-for-service to value-oriented payment. By improving the efficiency of health care through population health management, organizations can effectively pursue seemingly discrepant business incentives. At the same time, investing in new infrastructure for quality and value can help organizations pursue their missions to improve health and address the important national priority of high health care costs.

ACKNOWLEDGMENTS

The authors are grateful to Emma Healy, who provided substantial support in preparation of this article.

REFERENCES

1. Mongan JJ, Ferris TG, Lee TH. Options for slowing the growth of health care costs. New England Journal of Medicine 2008;358(14):1509–14.
2. Tanguturi VK, Temin E, Yeh RW, et al. Clinical interventions to reduce preventable hospital readmission after percutaneous coronary intervention. Circ Cardiovasc Qual Outcomes 2016;9(5):600–4.
3. Hong CS, Abrams MK, Ferris TG. Toward increased adoption of complex care management. N Engl J Med 2014;371(6):491–3.
4. Levy S, Bagley N, Rajkumar R. Reform at risk: mandating participation in alternative payment plans. N Engl J Med 2018;378(18):1663–5.
5. National Health Expenditure Data. Available at: https://www.cms.gov/Research-Statistics-Data-and-Systems/Statistics-Trends-and-Reports/NationalHealthExpend Data/NationalHealthAccountsHistorical.html.
6. Catlin A, Cowan C. History of health spending in the United States, 1960-2013. Cent Medicare Medicaid Serv; 2015. Available at: https://www.cms.gov/Research-Statistics-Data-and-Systems/Statistics-Trends-and-Reports/National HealthExpendData/Downloads/HistoricalNHEPaper.pdf.
7. Papanicolas I, Woskie LR, Jha AK. Health care spending in the United States and other high-income countries. JAMA 2018;319(10):1024–39.
8. The Effect of Health Care Cost Growth on the U.S. Economy. Office of the Assistant Secretary for Planning and Evaluation, U.S. Department of Health and

Human Services. Available at: https://aspe.hhs.gov/system/files/pdf/75441/report.pdf.

9. Khera R, Valero-Elizondo J, Okunrintemi V, et al. Association of out-of-pocket annual health expenditures with financial hardship in low-income adults with atherosclerotic cardiovascular disease in the United States. JAMA Cardiol 2018;3(8):729–38.

10. Dieleman JL, Squires E, Bui AL, et al. Factors associated with increases in US health care spending, 1996-2013. JAMA 2017;318(17):1668–78.

11. Blavin F. Association between the 2014 Medicaid expansion and US Hospital finances. JAMA 2016;316(14):1475–83.

12. Trends affecting hospitals and health systems. Available at: https://www.aha.org/guidesreports/2018-05-22-trendwatch-chartbook-2018. Accessed August 25, 2019.

13. Ly DP, Cutler DM. Factors of U.S. hospitals associated with improved profit margins: an observational study. J Gen Intern Med 2018;33(7):1020–7.

14. Cosgrove T. Value-based health care is inevitable and that's good. Harv Bus Rev 2013. Available at: https://hbr.org/2013/09/value-based-health-care-is-inevitable-and-thats-good. Accessed August 25, 2019.

15. Jain SH. 6 habits of high value health care organizations. Forbes; 2016. Available at: https://www.forbes.com/sites/sachinjain/2016/04/13/what-is-value-in-health-care-really-six-principles-from-organizations-bringing-value-to-patients/#730fdf125ad4.

16. Lee TH. Turning value-based health care into a real business model. NEJM Catal 2016. Available at: https://catalyst.nejm.org/turning-value-based-health-care-into-a-real-business-model/.

17. MGH mission. Available at: https://www.massgeneral.org/news/assets/PDF/HTLInsert020317.pdf. Accessed August 25, 2019.

18. Chung B, Brown A, Moreno G, et al. Implementing community engagement as a mission at the David Geffen School of Medicine at the University of California, Los Angeles. J Health Care Poor Underserved 2016;27(1):8–21.

19. Medicare to award contracts for demonstration projects to improve care for beneficiaries with high medical costs. Available at: https://innovation.cms.gov/Files/Migrated-Medicare-Demonstration-x/CMHCB_Press_Release.pdf. Accessed August 25, 2019.

20. Pioneer ACO model. Available at: https://innovation.cms.gov/initiatives/Pioneer-ACO-Model/. Accessed August 25, 2019.

21. Muhlestein D, Saunders R, Richards R, et al. Recent progress in the value journey: growth of ACOs and value-based payment models in 2018. Health Affairs Blog 2018. Available at: https://www.healthaffairs.org/do/10.1377/hblog2018 0810.481968/full/.

22. Shinkman R. Physician frustration and fear of MACRA. NEJM Catal 2016. Available at: https://catalyst.nejm.org/physician-frustration-fear-macra/.

Population Health and Academic Medical Centers
High Cost Meets High Efficiency

Sarah J. Conway, MD*, Scott A. Berkowitz, MD, MBA

KEYWORDS

- Population health • Academic medical centers • Value-based care
- Accountable care • Care coordination

KEY POINTS

- Academic medical centers (AMCs) have traditionally followed a tripartite mission of clinical care, research, and education with less focus on population health and value-based care.
- AMCs may have to expand their primary care footprints to serve a greater population. This expansion will provide them with needed patient volumes for their hospitals and training programs, and prioritize care delivery in the highest-value location.
- Changes in governance and leadership structures, health information technology advancements, and investments in care coordination are needed to succeed in achieving population health aims.

BACKGROUND

With the passage of the Affordable Care Act (ACA), there has been a shift in the way health care is delivered, prioritizing value and managing the health of populations.[1] With the transition to a population health–focused framework, the role for academic medical centers (AMCs) within care delivery is less certain. In the past, AMCs have followed a tripartite mission of clinical care, research, and education. However, nowhere embedded within those pillars is necessarily a prioritization of value; AMCs have historically been known for their organizational complexity and high overhead.[1]

In order to succeed in this new health care landscape, AMCs are at a precipice of change. AMCs will need to increasingly embrace interdisciplinary structures, achieve greater organizational nimbleness and flexibility, develop sophisticated knowledge management and communication capabilities, design financial incentives to align with population health priorities, and create robust information systems to support

Disclosure: The authors have nothing to disclose.
Johns Hopkins University School of Medicine, 733 North Broadway, Miller Research Building G45, Baltimore, MD 21205, USA
* Corresponding author.
E-mail address: sjc@jhmi.edu

Prim Care Clin Office Pract 46 (2019) 631–640
https://doi.org/10.1016/j.pop.2019.07.010
0095-4543/19/© 2019 Elsevier Inc. All rights reserved.

activities.[2] This change will necessitate reevaluation of how AMCs have traditionally operated. However, rather than abandoning their traditional priorities, they may find that reframing and reprioritizing are what is needed to endure and thrive within this changing landscape.

THE ROLE OF THE ACADEMIC MEDICAL CENTER

Embedded within the tripartite mission is the notion that AMCs lead research and discovery. They are the engine for biomedical advancement and receive significant funding from government and private sources to achieve these aims. Because of their novel clinical programs and concentrated expertise, AMCs also provide tertiary and quaternary care for a wide catchment area that necessarily feeds their research and discovery missions. In addition, AMCs are often so-called safety-net hospitals for patients with limited options because of complexity of care or socioeconomic circumstances. The patients served often have a high burden of chronic illness, substance abuse, mental illness, poverty, and other barriers to accessing care.[3]

Because of the unique position held by AMCs, the concept of Healthcare Innovation Zones (HIZs) was proposed around the time of the ACA and championed by the Association of American Medical Colleges.[4,5] The HIZ Pilot Act of 2009 (HR 3664) was introduced to the House of Representatives, intended for incorporation into the Center for Medicare and Medicaid Innovation.[6,7] The program was to include hospitals, health systems, insurers, group practitioners, and individual practitioners and allow them to design and test regionally specific integrated care delivery systems designed to improve the quality and control the cost of health care.[6] Each HIZ was to include an AMC that would be able to facilitate the rapid testing and evaluation of new delivery models while training the next generation of professionals to move the novel systems forward.[5] This bill did not move forward through the House, but does outline a framework that builds on the AMC framework and leverages its multifaceted mission to push toward the triple aim.

INHERENT TENSIONS OF ACADEMIC MEDICAL CENTERS AND POPULATION HEALTH: MAINTAINING THE TRIPARTITE MISSION

Although AMCs thrive on innovation, many of the inherent features that position them well in this arena limit their success in a value-based system. These features include a culture driven by specialties and use of novel, often more expensive, therapeutics. In order to support these specialties and investments in therapeutics and to sustain their training programs, AMCs need to retain revenues associated with maintaining patient clinical volumes. However, in value-based care models, these volumes may fundamentally be at risk. There is an increasing shift of routine or common care to lower-cost settings[8] in which trainees are often not present and that are away from where infrastructure and equipment investments have already been made. Examples include low-risk endoscopy and obstetric ultrasonography. In addition, many payers and competing health systems channel patients away from AMCs and exclude them from their networks because of the high cost of care and desire to retain their patients in the network.[8]

AMCs' current funding models and incentive alignment continue to support the system that has historically been in place. Changing those incentive systems is not easy given the decentralized structure of most AMCs with autonomous departments and more superficial clinical integration. Thus, although many AMCs have joined value-based health care programs, only a handful previously joined the higher-risk Pioneer Accountable Care Organizations (ACOs) or bundled payment demonstrations in part because of this tension. Many have focused instead on the Medicare Shared Savings Program (MSSP) upside only contracts. As the number of MSSP ACOs has increased from 333 to 432 between 2014 to 2016, the percentage of teaching hospitals in these ACOs has similarly increased from 18% to 28%.[9]

This article reviews the inherent tensions in place for each of the AMC pillars (clinical care, research, and education) and identifies opportunities for modification to fit the evolving value-based, population health framework.

CLINICAL CARE

AMCs traditionally fulfill 3 clinical roles: comprehensive population health manager for the local community, regional referral center for complex care, and national/international referral center for select subspecialties.[8] Often located in economically and socially disadvantaged areas, the population health manager role often manifests as provision of significant charity care.[1] AMCs comprise 6% of hospitals nationwide but provide 41% of hospital-based charity medical care.[10] Beyond this local community, AMCs have focused on development of their specialty and subspecialty services. For these, patients are often sent for a single-encounter diagnosis rather than long-term continuity of care.[3,11] With high fixed costs associated with investments in cutting-edge medical equipment, facilities, and personnel, hospitals have historically focused on maintaining the specialty referrals and high hospital occupancy rates.[12]

Opportunity

Health in the population health framework expands on the first clinical role as population health manager. This role extends beyond direct provision of clinical care to include wellness, preventive care, diagnosis, and management of disease.[1] The focus necessarily shifts to avoidance of acute care settings, which have previously been the financial drivers for AMCs. In this framework, AMCs must shift focus from cutting-edge facilities and specialty efforts to focus on population health programs. This focus includes an integrated primary care network to deliver preventive health; investments in low-cost, community-based treatment venues for acute and chronic care; patient engagement programs for lower-risk population management; and high-touch care management programs for complex and expensive patients.[12] Montefiore Medical Center has embraced this population health model with an integrated primary care network that leverages health information technology (IT) and high-risk patient programming through community partnerships. Their efforts have proved successful under high-risk Pioneer ACO contract.[13,14] Several AMCs have developed integrated behavioral health models to support their populations. UCLA advanced an integrated behavioral health program incorporating mental health providers into their primary care practices. They tripled the number of patients receiving behavioral health resources (4% to 13%) in 3 years with a 13% reduction in emergency department use.[15]

To maintain subspecialty care volumes while reducing hospitalizations for care that could be provided in a lower-acuity setting, there are opportunities to serve a wider catchment through an expanded primary care footprint and consolidate expensive clinical care resources through regionalization.[1,16] The resultant economies of scale and expertise provide tertiary and quaternary care for a broader community.[1] University of Virginia Health System has partnered with payers and providers to create regional systems that provide community-based care allowing patients to reap the benefits of AMC expertise while remaining close to home.[8] They train the workforce and feed them into the network. Providers retain their faculty appointments to preserve ties to the mother institution and allow access to ongoing training. The core clinical department can also provide community backup as needed. These partnerships are locally governed by agreed-on operating principles determined by the regional needs. Ultimately this allows patients to reap the benefits of AMC expertise while remaining close to home.

Further opportunities exist to overcome historically autonomous departments to pursue true clinical integration and coordination.[17] Several AMCs have begun this process of breaking down silos with development of service lines: coordinated collection of health care services that provide patients with a central access point to receive treatment across multiple disciplines, care providers, care sites, and time.[18] The goal is to create coordinated, high-quality, value-based care that standardizes care processes and offers a competitive advantage in the respective specialty area. UMass Memorial Health Care established a heart and vascular service line. Key success factors for that process included dedicated physician and administrative leadership enabled by financial support from the health system; clear accountability and authority over service line clinical programs, operations, finances, and staff; colocalization of faculty, personnel, and facilities; integration of education and training with weekly case-based conferences and cross-training; and multidisciplinary system improvement teams.[18]

Tying into the other parts of the tripartite mission, AMCs can innovate, study, and disseminate these various community interventions and expansion models to advance the fund of knowledge around population health.

RESEARCH

AMCs have long been drivers of innovation in health care and have developed academic systems in line with this goal. Promotion and advancement within AMCs is typically focused on publications, grant support, and scholarly reputation.[3,11] There is a historically long process for clinical innovation to make its way to the bedside. Faculty members are often funded with external grants with lower clinical effort often tailored to a narrow population of patients that supports their research. This structure limits the clinical incentive alignment opportunities for providers.[17] However, this research funding is increasingly at risk as federal support dollars decline and clinical margins for support shrink.[19] The cost of research now exceeds the dollars available to support it.[19]

Opportunity

AMCs in the population health framework need not abandon their commitment to research. However, they may need to adjust the research priorities, increasing focus on areas that have traditionally been undersupported, such as behavioral science, public health–related research, informatics, management sciences, and health services research.[2] There are opportunities to advance implementation science with the testing and evaluation of new delivery models.[17] These evaluations will largely be quality improvement studies and may not allow for the gold standard double-blind randomized control trials. However, there are options for rigorous evaluations in the quality improvement context, such as difference-in-difference analyses. The goal is rapid and continuous process improvement to support successes in advanced and adaptive care delivery models.[3]

Tested initiatives may range from value-based quality improvement initiatives, such as the Choosing Wisely campaign,[16,20] to whole-scale evaluations of major policy cross-continuum implementations.[21] In the big-data era with increasing unification of electronic medical record (EMR) platforms and new technologies available to engage patients (ie, mobile devices), there are opportunities to be learning health systems.[19] In addition, there are opportunities to collaborate with diverse partners for research, including nonacademic institutions, industry, and governmental entities.

In addition, as AMCs work to align clinical incentives with those that meet their greater population health metrics, they are increasingly offering alternative career tracks. These clinical tracks allow for promotion based on clinical expertise rather than research success. High-quality physicians who are primarily focused on care delivery are well suited to implement novel changes in care delivery, can be adequately incentivized to achieve quality and efficiency metrics, and can maintain the clinical enterprise needed to sustain the more specialized parts of the system. For those faculty that remain within the traditional research track, AMCs will need to redefine success as it relates to scientific and societal impact rather than strictly funding or number of articles published.[19]

EDUCATION

AMCs train most allopathic medical students and half of the nation's residents and interns.[2] They are thus primarily responsible for crafting the future health care workforce. Traditional medical education has focused on pathology and pathophysiology of disease and less on care delivery and high-value care. The funding for teaching health systems has supported the propagation of an inefficient system. Providers are educated in a silo with limited integration with other members of the care delivery workforce. Several institutions have created collaborative models for research across disciplines inclusive of medicine, nursing, and public health, such as the Leonard Davis Institute of Health Economics at the University of Pennsylvania[22] and the Welch Center for Prevention, Epidemiology, and Clinical Research at Johns Hopkins University.[23]

Opportunities

Training and education programs will need to be adjusted to adequately train the workforce of the future to practice within the population health framework. This adjustment includes leveraging university affiliations to redesign care delivery, drawing on insights from health and behavioral economics, psychology, sociology, policy and management, industrial engineering, and computer science.[19] AMCs will need to focus on increasing interprofessional education and broadening their areas of focus. Increasingly there are courses targeted at teaching basic principles of care transformation and clinical integration. Many of these have focused on individuals who have already completed their professional training but are increasingly present in medical school curricula. A High Value Practice Academic Alliance is further advancing this work, bringing institutions together to share the methodology and the learnings.[24]

As AMCs look to expand their footprint to adequately feed their clinical enterprise, they should incorporate the needs of their medical training programs into the expansion calculations. The local community population is needed to support primary care and core residency programs. The regional and national volumes are often required for fellowships and specialized programs such as neurosurgery.[8] University of Michigan and Johns Hopkins University are two AMCs that have used the training program requirements to drive estimates on the size of their clinical expansions.[8] Michigan projected it needs 400,000 covered lives within its primary service area and 3 million to 4 million covered lives overall to ensure adequate specialty volume to meet its educational needs.[8] In order to achieve these target network sizes, the institutions have worked on expanding their physician networks, their affiliations and partnerships, their employer/payer relationships, and their fully integrated partnerships (ie, acquisitions).[8] University of Michigan has also embraced potential disrupters, such as partnering with CVS Minute Clinics for virtual care capabilities with telemedicine, patient portals, and smart phone applications to improve access.[8]

WHAT IS NEEDED FOR ACADEMIC MEDICAL CENTER SUCCESS

As AMCs chart the path toward success in a new population health framework, it is valuable to identify what success looks like and the key changes needed. The key factors evaluated include quality performance, resource use, and cost. These factors are often features of value-based contracts, such as ACOs (federal payer or commercial), bundled payment programs, and global payment agreements such as the Global Budget Revenue in Maryland. Performing well on these metrics aligns with financial incentives under these various alternative payment models. Those proceeds, when received, can be used to fund initiatives to support ongoing population health efforts for existing or new populations.

AMCs need to make several changes in order to succeed and meet these evolving value-based metrics. The key areas include leadership and governance, robust IT and analytics, and care coordination and management. Core to all these is a change in the institutional culture to allow them to quickly adapt to a constantly changing environment. This cultural change is not to be underestimated and will likely be a lengthy and complex process for each AMC. The changes in institutional culture should increase teamwork, commitment to a learning health system, continuous improvement, accountability, and patient-centeredness.[2]

Governance and Leadership

Core to driving the needed culture change is a commitment by leadership and a governance structure that supports the value-based and population-based priorities. The corporate organizational structure needs to allow for responsiveness and quick action to be more responsive to community needs.[2] This structure can benefit from an accountable leader who reports directly to a chief executive optimally overseeing both the university and clinical delivery entities.[3] This executive needs to manage tensions that will inevitably arise between accountable and academic care.[12] Population health innovations may erode profitability of existing previously autonomous departments for the benefit of the greater organization and community.[12]

The population health infrastructure will need to be responsible for internal accounting with a dedicated funds flow and an ability to manage budgeting in alignment with priorities.[2,12] Each AMC will need to determine where these funds should come from both initially and over time. For example, initial investments may need to be made by the health system and ultimately supplanted by value-based reimbursements. Alternative structures may include a tax on care delivery revenues or another revenue-generating approach to dedicate for population health activities. Various sources of government dollars may support these activities, such as care management fees provided through Comprehensive Primary Care Plus programs[25] or infrastructure dollars for care coordination provided to Maryland hospitals as part of the Maryland All-Payer Model.[26]

Once funding is secured and leadership organization structure is in place, there needs to be a capacity for continuous performance measurement and performance improvement. AMCs will need to incorporate best practices. These best practices may be identified from within their organizations or externally from other AMCs as well as other nonacademic organizations.[2] Strategic review processes that incorporate these best practices along with community and population data are key to ongoing success.[27]

Health Information Technology

AMCs have access to robust information systems that allow integration of data from EMREMRs, claims history, administrative data, and other data sources. The analytical power and risk prediction models being developed are key to success as a learning health system. They will drive precision medicine in the population health context. These data are needed to facilitate monitoring of quality measures, create decision-support tools, and develop care coordination tools.[16]

These data must be readily accessible to convert real-time population health information into care management programs. They facilitate patient-centered strategies and create opportunities for study and continuous process improvement.[3] AMCs can benefit from economies of scale for their IT infrastructure investments.[3] However, as they expand to new footprints and incorporate community providers, they will need to bridge disparate Health IT platforms, which may limit their ability to measure and monitor quality and harmonize various EMR-based interventions.[16]

Care Coordination

Coordinated care is key to managing populations. Health IT infrastructure can monitor quality and safety metrics to track performance in this realm. However, execution of this directive requires a higher level of care team integration with multidisciplinary representation to address the various factors that contribute to health outcomes for a population. There is an evolving body of literature on care coordination best practices,[28] but execution is key to these interventions and continual monitoring and modification are needed to ensure they are achieving stated aims.

Adequate access has been difficult for AMCs with limited focus on primary care access points and notoriously long wait times for specialty appointments. Expansion of access will be part of growing the primary care footprint and may come from strategic

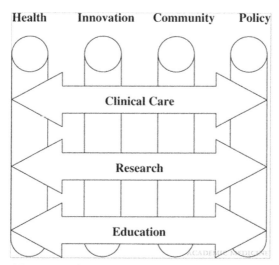

Fig. 1. A conceptual framework for academic health centers. (*From* Borden WB, Mushlin AI, Gordon JE, et al. A new conceptual framework for academic health centers. Acad Med. 2015;90:570; with permission.)

alignment with community partners rather than organic growth. These partners will need to have a shared sense of vision and support the strategic priorities[16] but offer a quicker way to scale and bring on more clinically focused providers. Partnerships can expand beyond addition of physician groups and may include opportunities for integration across the continuum with postacute care providers as well.[16,29] For internal growth opportunities, offering a clinical track as well as generalist specialists will also increase needed access.

Health systems with a history or ability to manage risk will be well suited for this challenge, possibly through prior experience of owning a managed care plan or success under value-based arrangements. They will have demonstrated an ability to align provider and care team incentives with defined value-based goals.

SUMMARY

Academic medicine is at an inflection point with the changing priorities of health care to focus more on population health. However, to survive in this new model of care, the AMC tripartite mission need not be abandoned. Instead, those guiding pillars will need to be reworked into a new framework that prioritizes management of populations, integration, adaptability, and rapid learning. Borden and colleagues[1] propose a new conceptual framework to expand on the triple mission for AMCs along 4 new dimensions: health, innovation, community, and policy (**Fig. 1**). The field remains ripe for study and evaluation and society will continue to look to academic institutions to drive this work.

To complete this change, AMCs will have to undergo the hard work of culture change. This change will be facilitated by restructuring governance and organizational structures to fund and support the population health view. AMCs will need to invest in care coordination and fund health IT enhancements to support this work. Learning health systems will need to continuously evolve to meet the changing needs of the populations served.

REFERENCES

1. Borden WB, Mushlin AI, Gordon JE, et al. A new conceptual framework for academic health centers. Acad Med 2015;90(5):569–73.
2. Envisioning the future of academic health centers final report of the commonwealth fund task force on academic health centers. 2003. Available at: www.cmwf.org. Accessed November 26, 2018.
3. Berkowitz SA, Pahira JJ. Accountable care organization readiness and academic medical centers. Acad Med 2014;89(9):1210–5.
4. AAMC President advocates for Healthcare Innovation Zones (HIZs). AAMC Washington Highlights. 2010. Available at: https://www.aamc.org/advocacy/washhigh/highlights2010/162196/aamc_president_advocates_for_healthcare_innovation_zones.html. Accessed December 31, 2018.
5. AAMC. How Healthcare Innovation Zones (HIZs) can leverage the best of American medicine. Available at: www.aamc.org/newsroom. Accessed December 9, 2018.
6. Kirch DG. The healthcare innovation zone. JAMA 2010;303(9):874.
7. Schwartz A. H.R.3664 - Healthcare Innovation Zone Pilot Act of 2009. 111th Congress (2009-2010). 2009. Available at: https://www.congress.gov/bill/111th-congress/house-bill/3664. Accessed December 9, 2018.
8. The Blue Ridge Academic Health Group. Synchronizing the academic health center clinical enterprise and education mission in changing environments.

2016. Available at: http://whsc.emory.edu/blueridge/publications/archive/Blue Ridge-2016.pdf. Accessed December 9, 2018.

9. AAMC. AAMC Analysis of Medicare Shared Savings Program (MSSP) Research Identifiable Files (RIF) 2014 through 2016 2018.

10. Academic Medicine. Where patients turn for hope. Available at: https://members. aamc.org/eweb/upload/Academic Medicine Where Patients Turn for Hope.pdf. Accessed November 26, 2018.

11. Kastor JA. Accountable care organizations at academic medical centers. N Engl J Med 2010. https://doi.org/10.1056/NEJMp1002530.

12. Stein D, Chen C, Ackerly DC. Disruptive innovation in academic medical centers. Acad Med 2015;90(5):594–8.

13. Foreman S. Montefiore Medical Center in the Bronx, New York: improving health in an urban community. Acad Med 2004. https://doi.org/10.1097/00001888-200412000-00007.

14. Bachrach D, Pfister H, Wallis K, et al. Addressing patients' social needs: an emerging business care for provider investment. New York: Commonw Fund; 2014.

15. Clarke RMA, Jeffrey J, Grossman M, et al. Delivering on accountable care: lessons from a behavioral health program to improve access and outcomes. Health Aff (Millwood) 2016;35(8):1487–93.

16. Berkowitz SA, Ishii L, Schulz J, et al. Academic medical centers forming accountable care organizations and partnering with community providers. Acad Med 2016;91(3):328–32.

17. Berkowitz SA, Miller ED. Accountable care at academic medical centers-lessons from Johns Hopkins. N Engl J Med 2011;364(7):e12.

18. Phillips RA, Cyr J, Keaney JF, et al. Creating and maintaining a successful service line in an academic medical center at the dawn of value-based care: lessons learned from the heart and vascular service line at UMass Memorial Health Care. Acad Med 2015;90(10):1340–6.

19. Dzau VJ, Cho A, ElLaissi W, et al. Transforming academic health centers for an uncertain future. N Engl J Med 2013. https://doi.org/10.1056/NEJMp1302374.

20. Choosing wisely web site. Available at: http://www.choosingwisely.org/. Accessed November 21, 2018.

21. Berkowitz SA, Parashuram S, Rowan K, et al. Association of a care coordination model with health care costs and utilization. JAMA Netw Open 2018;1(7): e184273.

22. Leonard Davis Institute of Health Economics. Available at: https://ldi.upenn.edu/. Accessed December 27, 2018.

23. The Welch Center for Prevention. Epidemiology, and clinical research - Centers and Institutes - Research - Johns Hopkins Bloomberg School of Public Health. Available at: https://www.jhsph.edu/research/centers-and-institutes/welch-center-for-prevention-epidemiology-and-clinical-research/index.html. Accessed December 27, 2018.

24. HVPAA • High Value Practice Academic Alliance. Available at: http://hvpaa.org/. Accessed December 27, 2018.

25. Centers for Medicare and Medicaid Services. Comprehensive primary care plus. Available at: https://innovation.cms.gov/initiatives/comprehensive-primary-care-plus/. Accessed December 28, 2018.

26. Centers for Medicare & Medicaid Services. Maryland all-payer model to deliver better care and lower costs. 2014. Available at: https://www.cms.gov/Newsroom/

MediaReleaseDatabase/Fact-Sheets/2014-Fact-sheets-items/2014-01-10.html. Accessed December 21, 2016.

27. Conway SJ, Himmelrich S, Feeser SA, et al. Strategic review process for an accountable care organization and emerging accountable care best practices. Popul Health Manag 2018;21(5):357–65.

28. Brown RS, Peikes D, Peterson G, et al. Six features of medicare coordinated care demonstration programs that cut hospital admissions of high-risk patients. Health Aff 2012;31(6):1156–66.

29. Conway SJ, Parekh AK, Hughes AH, et al. Next steps in improving healthcare value: PostAcute care transitions: developing a skilled nursing facility collaborative within an academic health system. J Hosp Med 2019;14(3):174–7.

UNITED STATES POSTAL SERVICE ® Statement of Ownership, Management, and Circulation (All Periodicals Publications Except Requester Publications)

1. Publication Title	2. Publication Number	3. Filing Date
PRIMARY CARE: CLINICS IN OFFICE PRACTICE	044 – 690	9/18/2019

4. Issue Frequency	5. Number of Issues Published Annually	6. Annual Subscription Price
MAR, JUN, SEP, DEC	4	$246.00

7. Complete Mailing Address of Known Office of Publication (Not printer) (Street, city, county, state, and ZIP+4®)

ELSEVIER INC.
230 Park Avenue, Suite 800
New York, NY 10169

Contact Person
STEPHEN R. BUSHING
Telephone (Include area code)
215-239-3688

8. Complete Mailing Address of Headquarters or General Business Office of Publisher (Not printer)

ELSEVIER INC.
230 Park Avenue, Suite 800
New York, NY 10169

9. Full Names and Complete Mailing Addresses of Publisher, Editor, and Managing Editor (Do not leave blank)

Publisher (Name and complete mailing address)

TAYLOR BALL, ELSEVIER INC.
1600 JOHN F KENNEDY BLVD. SUITE 1800
PHILADELPHIA, PA 19103-2899

Editor (Name and complete mailing address)

JESSICA MCCOOL, ELSEVIER INC.
1600 JOHN F KENNEDY BLVD. SUITE 1800
PHILADELPHIA, PA 19103-2899

Managing Editor (Name and complete mailing address)

PATRICK MANLEY, ELSEVIER INC.
1600 JOHN F KENNEDY BLVD. SUITE 1800
PHILADELPHIA, PA 19103-2899

10. Owner (Do not leave blank. If the publication is owned by a corporation, give the name and address of the corporation immediately followed by the names and addresses of all stockholders owning or holding 1 percent or more of the total amount of stock. If not owned by a corporation, give the names and addresses of the individual owners. If owned by a partnership or other unincorporated firm, give its name and address as well as those of each individual owner. If the publication is published by a nonprofit organization, give its name and address.)

Full Name	Complete Mailing Address
WHOLLY OWNED SUBSIDIARY OF REED/ELSEVIER, US HOLDINGS	1600 JOHN F KENNEDY BLVD. SUITE 1800 PHILADELPHIA, PA 19103-2899

11. Known Bondholders, Mortgagees, and Other Security Holders Owning or Holding 1 Percent or More of Total Amount of Bonds, Mortgages, or Other Securities. If none, check box. ► ☐ None

Full Name	Complete Mailing Address
N/A	

12. Tax Status (For completion by nonprofit organizations authorized to mail at nonprofit rates) (Check one)
The purpose, function, and nonprofit status of this organization and the exempt status for federal income tax purposes:
☒ Has Not Changed During Preceding 12 Months
☐ Has Changed During Preceding 12 Months (Publisher must submit explanation of change with this statement)

PS Form 3526, July 2014 (Page 1 of 4 (see instructions page 4)) PSN 7530-01-000-9931 PRIVACY NOTICE: See our privacy policy on www.usps.com.

---

13. Publication Title	14. Issue Date for Circulation Data Below
PRIMARY CARE: CLINICS IN OFFICE PRACTICE	JUNE 2019

15. Extent and Nature of Circulation			Average No. Copies Each Issue During Preceding 12 Months	No. Copies of Single Issue Published Nearest to Filing Date
a. Total Number of Copies (Net press run)			98	87
b. Paid Circulation (By Mail and Outside the Mail)	(1)	Mailed Outside-County Paid Subscriptions Stated on PS Form 3541 (Include paid distribution above nominal rate, advertiser's proof copies, and exchange copies)	36	44
	(2)	Mailed In-County Paid Subscriptions Stated on PS Form 3541 (Include paid distribution above nominal rate, advertiser's proof copies, and exchange copies)	0	0
	(3)	Paid Distribution Outside the Mails Including Sales Through Dealers and Carriers, Street Vendors, Counter Sales, and Other Paid Distribution Outside USPS®	12	14
	(4)	Paid Distribution by Other Classes of Mail Through the USPS (e.g. First-Class Mail®)	0	0
c. Total Paid Distribution (Sum of 15b (1), (2), (3), and (4))		►	48	58
d. Free or Nominal Rate Distribution (By Mail and Outside the Mail)	(1)	Free or Nominal Rate Outside-County Copies included on PS Form 3541	34	13
	(2)	Free or Nominal Rate In-County Copies Included on PS Form 3541	0	0
	(3)	Free or Nominal Rate Copies Mailed at Other Classes Through the USPS (e.g. First-Class Mail)	0	0
	(4)	Free or Nominal Rate Distribution Outside the Mail (Carriers or other means)	0	0
e. Total Free or Nominal Rate Distribution (Sum of 15d (1), (2), (3) and (4))		►	34	13
f. Total Distribution (Sum of 15c and 15e)		►	82	71
g. Copies not Distributed (See Instructions to Publishers #4 (page #3))		►	16	16
h. Total (Sum of 15f and g)		►	98	87
i. Percent Paid (15c divided by 15f times 100)		►	58.54%	81.69%

* If you are claiming electronic copies, go to line 16 on page 3. If you are not claiming electronic copies, skip to line 17 on page 3.

16. Electronic Copy Circulation	Average No. Copies Each Issue During Preceding 12 Months	No. Copies of Single Issue Published Nearest to Filing Date
a. Paid Electronic Copies ►		
b. Total Paid Print Copies (Line 15c) + Paid Electronic Copies (Line 16a) ►		
c. Total Print Distribution (Line 15f) + Paid Electronic Copies (Line 16a) ►		
d. Percent Paid (Both Print & Electronic Copies) (16b divided by 16c × 100) ►		

☒ I certify that 50% of all my distributed copies (electronic and print) are paid above a nominal price.

17. Publication of Statement of Ownership

☒ If the publication is a general publication, publication of this statement is required. Will be printed in the DECEMBER 2019 issue of this publication. ☐ Publication not required.

18. Signature and Title of Editor, Publisher, Business Manager, or Owner

STEPHEN R. BUSHING - INVENTORY DISTRIBUTION CONTROL MANAGER

Date 9/18/2019

I certify that all information furnished on this form is true and complete. I understand that anyone who furnishes false or misleading information on this form or who omits material or information requested on the form may be subject to criminal sanctions (including civil penalties).

PS Form 3526, July 2014 (Page 3 of 4) PRIVACY NOTICE: See our privacy policy on www.usps.com

Printed and bound by CPI Group (UK) Ltd, Croydon, CR0 4YY

03/10/2024

01040484-0018